Sleep and the Heart

Editor

RAMI N. KHAYAT

SLEEP MEDICINE CLINICS

www.sleep.theclinics.com

Consulting Editor
TEOFILO LEE-CHIONG Jr

June 2017 • Volume 12 • Number 2

ELSEVIER

1600 John F. Kennedy Boulevard • Suite 1800 • Philadelphia, Pennsylvania, 19103-2899

http://www.theclinics.com

SLEEP MEDICINE CLINICS Volume 12, Number 2
June 2017, ISSN 1556-407X, ISBN-13: 978-0-323-53031-6

Editor: Katie Pfaff
Developmental Editor: Donald Mumford

Sleep Medicine Clinics (ISSN 1556-407X) is published quarterly by Elsevier Inc., 360 Park Avenue South, New York, NY 10010-1710. Months of issue are March, June, September and December. Business and Editorial Offices: 1600 John F. Kennedy Blvd., Ste. 1800, Philadelphia, PA 19103-2899. Customer Service Office: 3251 Riverport Lane, Maryland Heights, MO 63043. Periodicals postage paid at New York, NY and additional mailing offices. Subscription prices are $203.00 per year (US individuals), $100.00 (US students), $476.00 (US institutions), $244.00 (Canadian and international individuals), $135.00 (Canadian and international students), $540.00 (Canadian institutions) and $529.00 (International institutions). Foreign air speed delivery is included in all *Clinics* subscription prices. All prices are subject to change without notice. **POSTMASTER:** Send change of address to *Sleep Medicine Clinics*, Elsevier Health Sciences Division, Subscription Customer Service, 3251 Riverport Lane, Maryland Heights, MO 63043. Customer Service: **Tel: 1-800-654-2452 (U.S. and Canada); 314-447-8871 (outside U.S. and Canada). Fax: 314-447-8029. E-mail: journalscustomerservice-usa@elsevier.com (for print support); journalsonline support-usa@elsevier.com (for online support).**

Reprints. For copies of 100 or more of articles in this publication, please contact the Commercial Reprints Department, Elsevier Inc., 360 Park Avenue South, New York, NY 10010-1710. Tel.: 212-633-3874; Fax: 212-633-3820; E-mail: reprints@elsevier.com.

Sleep Medicine Clinics is covered in *MEDLINE/PubMed (Index Medicus)*.

PROGRAM OBJECTIVE

The goal of *Sleep Clinics of North America* is to keep practicing physicians up to date with current clinical practice by providing timely articles reviewing the state of the art in patient care.

TARGET AUDIENCE

All practicing physicians and other healthcare professionals.

LEARNING OBJECTIVES

Upon completion of this activity, participants will be able to:
1. Review the effects of insomnia and other sleep disorders on cardiovascular conditions.
2. Discuss sleep and cardiovascular problems in children.
3. Recognize possible treatments for sleep apnea in patients with cardiovascular conditions.

ACCREDITATION

The Elsevier Office of Continuing Medical Education (EOCME) is accredited by the Accreditation Council for Continuing Medical Education (ACCME) to provide continuing medical education for physicians.

The EOCME designates this enduring material for a maximum of 15 *AMA PRA Category 1 Credit*(s)™. Physicians should claim only the credit commensurate with the extent of their participation in the activity.

All other health care professionals requesting continuing education credit for this enduring material will be issued a certificate of participation.

DISCLOSURE OF CONFLICTS OF INTEREST

The EOCME assesses conflict of interest with its instructors, faculty, planners, and other individuals who are in a position to control the content of CME activities. All relevant conflicts of interest that are identified are thoroughly vetted by EOCME for fair balance, scientific objectivity, and patient care recommendations. EOCME is committed to providing its learners with CME activities that promote improvements or quality in healthcare and not a specific proprietary business or a commercial interest.

The planning committee, staff, authors and editors listed below have identified no financial relationships or relationships to products or devices they or their spouse/life partner have with commercial interest related to the content of this CME activity:

Rita Aouad, MD; M. Safwan Badr, MD; Thomas Bitter, MD; Anjali Fortna; Henrik Fox, MD; Simon Herkenrath, MD; Dieter Horstkotte, MD, PhD, FESC, FACCP; Behrouz Jafari, MD; Rami Kahwash, MD; Meena S. Khan, MD; Rami N. Khayat, MD; Olaf Oldenburg, MD; Grace R. Paul, MD; Katie Pfaff; Swaroop Pinto, MD; James A. Rowley, MD; Rajakumar Venkatesan; Katie Widmeier, Amy Williams.

The planning committee, staff, authors and editors listed below have identified financial relationships or relationships to products or devices they or their spouse/life partner have with commercial interest related to the content of this CME activity:

Robin Germany, MD has an employment affiliation with Respicardia Inc.
Teofilo Lee-Chiong Jr, MD is a consultant/advisor for Elsevier and CareCore International, has stock ownership in and an employment affiliation with Elsevier, and receieves royalties/patents from Lippincott; Oxford University Press; CreateSpace; and Wiley.
Winfried Randerath, MD is on the speakers' bureau for Heinen + Löwenstein; Philips; Weinmann; Inspire; and ResMed.

UNAPPROVED/OFF-LABEL USE DISCLOSURE

The EOCME requires CME faculty to disclose to the participants:
1. When products or procedures being discussed are off-label, unlabelled, experimental, and/or investigational (not US Food and Drug Administration [FDA] approved); and
2. Any limitations on the information presented, such as data that are preliminary or that represent ongoing research, interim analyses, and/or unsupported opinions. Faculty may discuss information about pharmaceutical agents that is outside of FDA-approved labelling. This information is intended solely for CME and is not intended to promote off-label use of these medications. If you have any questions, contact the medical affairs department of the manufacturer for the most recent prescribing information.

TO ENROLL

To enroll in the Sleep Medicines Clinic Continuing Medical Education program, call customer service at 1-800-654-2452 or sign up online at http://www.theclinics.com/home/cme. The CME program is available to subscribers for an additional annual fee of USD– $140.

METHOD OF PARTICIPATION

In order to claim credit, participants must complete the following:
1. Complete enrolment as indicated above.

2. Read the activity.
3. Complete the CME Test and Evaluation. Participants must achieve a score of 70% on the test. All CME Tests and Evaluations must be completed online.

CME INQUIRIES/SPECIAL NEEDS

For all CME inquiries or special needs, please contact elsevierCME@elsevier.com.

SLEEP MEDICINE CLINICS

ISSUES OF RELATED INTEREST

Clinics in Chest Medicine, Vol. 35, No. 3 (September 2014)
Sleep-Disordered Breathing: Beyond Obstructive Sleep Apnea
Carolyn M. D'Ambrosio, *Editor*
Available at: http://www.chestmed.theclinics.com/

THE CLINICS ARE AVAILABLE ONLINE!
Access your subscription at:
www.theclinics.com

Contributors

CONSULTING EDITOR

TEOFILO LEE-CHIONG Jr, MD
Professor of Medicine, National Jewish Health,
School of Medicine, University of Colorado
Denver, Denver, Colorado; Chief Medical
Liaison, Philips Respironics, Pennsylvania

EDITOR

RAMI N. KHAYAT, MD
Professor, Internal Medicine, Director, The
OSU Sleep Heart Program, Medical Director,
Respiratory Therapy, Division of Pulmonary,
Allergy, Critical Care, and Sleep Medicine,
Department of Internal Medicine, Davis Heart &
Lung Research Institute, The Ohio State
University, Columbus, Ohio

AUTHORS

RITA AOUAD, MD
Sleep Medicine Fellow, Division of Pulmonary,
Critical Care, and Sleep Medicine, Department
of Internal Medicine, The Ohio State University,
Columbus, Ohio

M. SAFWAN BADR, MD
Professor of Medicine, Division of Pulmonary,
Critical Care & Sleep Medicine, Harper
University Hospital, John D. Dingell VAMC,
Wayne State University School of Medicine,
Detroit, Michigan

THOMAS BITTER, MD
Clinic for Cardiology, Herz- und
Diabeteszentrum NRW, Ruhr-Universität
Bochum, Bad Oeynhausen, Germany

HENRIK FOX, MD
Clinic for Cardiology, Herz- und
Diabeteszentrum NRW, Ruhr-Universität
Bochum, Bad Oeynhausen, Germany

ROBIN GERMANY, MD
Clinical Assistant Professor of Medicine,
Cardiovascular Division, University of
Oklahoma College of Medicine, Oklahoma
City, Oklahoma

SIMON HERKENRATH, MD
Clinic for Pneumology and Allergology,
Centre of Sleep Medicine and Respiratory
Care, Bethanien Hospital, Institute of
Pneumology, University of Cologne,
Solingen, Germany

**DIETER HORSTKOTTE, MD, PhD, FESC,
FACCP**
Clinic for Cardiology, Herz- und
Diabeteszentrum NRW, Ruhr-Universität
Bochum, Bad Oeynhausen, Germany

BEHROUZ JAFARI, MD
Assistant Professor of Medicine,
Section of Pulmonary, Critical Care
and Sleep Medicine, School of Medicine,
University of California-Irvine, Irvine,
California; Director of Sleep Program,
VA Long Beach Healthcare System, Long
Beach, California

RAMI KAHWASH, MD
Associate Professor of Internal Medicine,
Section of Heart Failure and Transplant,
Division of Cardiovascular Medicine, Davis
Heart & Lung Research Institute, The Ohio
State University, Columbus, Ohio

MEENA S. KHAN, MD
Assistant Professor, Division of Pulmonary,
Critical Care, and Sleep Medicine,
Department of Internal Medicine and
Neurology, The Ohio State University,
Columbus, Ohio

RAMI N. KHAYAT, MD
Professor, Internal Medicine, Director, The
OSU Sleep Heart Program, Medical Director,
Respiratory Therapy, Division of Pulmonary,
Allergy, Critical Care, and Sleep Medicine,
Department of Internal Medicine, Davis Heart &
Lung Research Institute, The Ohio State
University, Columbus, Ohio

OLAF OLDENBURG, MD
Clinic for Cardiology, Herz- und
Diabeteszentrum NRW, Ruhr-Universität
Bochum, Bad Oeynhausen, Germany

GRACE R. PAUL, MD
Assistant Professor of Pediatrics, Division of
Pulmonary and Sleep Medicine, Nationwide
Children's Hospital, The Ohio State University,
Columbus, Ohio

SWAROOP PINTO, MD
Assistant Professor of Pediatrics, Division of
Pulmonary and Sleep Medicine, Nationwide
Children's Hospital, The Ohio State University,
Columbus, Ohio

WINFRIED RANDERATH, MD
Professor, Clinic for Pneumology and
Allergology, Centre of Sleep Medicine and
Respiratory Care, Bethanien Hospital, Institute
of Pneumology, University of Cologne,
Solingen, Germany

JAMES A. ROWLEY, MD
Professor of Medicine, Division of
Pulmonary, Critical Care & Sleep Medicine,
Harper University Hospital, Wayne State
University School of Medicine, Detroit,
Michigan

Contents

Different stages of sleep are associated with significant variability in cardiovascular function, which is mediated by marked changes in balance between 2 components of the autonomic system: parasympathetic and sympathetic. Autonomic control of circulation is essential in ensuring an adequate blood flow to vital organs through constant adjustments of arterial blood pressure, heart rate, and redistribution of blood flow. Fluctuations in components of the autonomic nervous system synchronize with electroencephalographic activity during arousal or different stages of sleep. As a result, these can lead to several cardiovascular consequences in those who have underlying heart disease or sleep-disordered breathing.

Sleep loss has negative impacts on quality of life, mood, cognitive function, and heath. Insomnia is linked to poor mood, increased use of health care resources, decreased quality of life, and possibly cardiovascular risk factors and disease. Studies have shown increase in cortisol levels, decreased immunity, and increased markers of sympathetic activity in sleep-deprived healthy subjects and those with chronic insomnia. The literature shows subjective complaints consistent with chronic insomnia and shortened sleep can be associated with development of diabetes, hypertension, and cardiovascular disease. This article explores the relationship between insufficient sleep and insomnia with these health conditions.

Subspecialty pediatric practice provides comprehensive medical care for a range of ages, from premature infants to children, and often includes adults with complex medical and surgical issues that warrant multidisciplinary care. Normal physiologic variations involving different body systems occur during sleep and these vary with age, stage of sleep, and underlying health conditions. This article is a concise review of the cardiovascular (CV) physiology and pathophysiology in children, sleep-disordered breathing (SDB) contributing to CV morbidity, congenital and acquired CV pathology resulting in SDB, and the relationship between SDB and CV morbidity in different clinical syndromes and systemic diseases in the expanded pediatric population.

Obstructive sleep apnea (OSA) is present in more than 50% of patients referred to cardiac rehabilitation units. However, it has been under-recognized in patients after stroke and heart failure. Those with concurrent OSA have a worse clinical course.

Early treatment of coexisting OSA with continuous positive airway pressure (CPAP) results in improved rehabilitation outcomes and quality of life. Possible mechanisms by which CPAP may improve recovery include decreased blood pressure fluctuations associated with apneas, and improved left ventricular function, cerebral blood flow, and oxygenation. Early screening and treatment of OSA should be integral components of patients entering cardiac rehabilitation units.

Sleep-disordered breathing (SDB) is a major health problem affecting much of the general population. Although SDB is responsible for rapid progression of heart failure (HF) and the worsening morbidity and mortality, advanced HF state is associated with accelerated development of SDB. In the face of recent developments in SDB treatment and availability of effective therapeutic options known to improve quality of life, exercise tolerance, and heart function, most HF patients with SDB are left unrecognized and untreated. This article provides an overview of SDB in HF with focus on practical approaches intended to facilitate screening and treatment.

Central sleep apnea and Cheyne-Stokes respiration are commonly observed breathing patterns during sleep in patients with congestive heart failure. Common risk factors are male gender, older age, presence of atrial fibrillation, and daytime hypocapnia. Proposed mechanisms include augmented peripheral and central chemoreceptor sensitivity, which increase ventilator instability during both wakefulness and sleep; diminished cerebrovascular reactivity and increased circulation time, which impair the normal buffering of $Paco_2$ and hydrogen ions and delay the detection of changes in $Paco_2$ during sleep; and rostral fluid shifts that predispose to hypocapnia.

Heart failure (HF) treatment remains complex and challenging, with current recommendations aiming at consideration and treatment of comorbidities in patients with HF. Sleep-disordered breathing (SDB) and arrhythmia come into play, as both are associated with quality of life deterioration, and morbidity and mortality increase in patients with HF. Interactions of these diseases are versatile and may appear intransparent in daily practice. Nevertheless, because of their importance for patients' condition and prognosis, SDB and arrhythmia individually, but also through interaction on one another, necessitate attention, following the fact that treatment is requested and desired considering latest research findings and outcomes.

Pathophysiologic components of upper airway obstruction, reduced tidal volume, and disturbed respiratory drive characterize sleep-disordered breathing. Positive airway pressure (PAP) devices address these components by stabilizing the upper airways (continuous PAP), applying air volumes and mandatory breaths (bilevel PAP), or counterbalancing ventilation (adaptive servoventilation). Although PAP therapies have been shown to improve breathing disturbances, daytime symptoms, and left ventricular function in obstructive sleep apnea and cardiovascular diseases, the effects on mortality are controversial, especially in heart failure and central sleep apnea. Optimal treatment is selected based on polysomnographic findings and symptoms, and applied based on the underlying pathophysiologic components.

Central sleep apnea is common in heart failure and contributes to morbidity and mortality. Symptoms are often similar to those associated with heart failure and a high index of suspicion is needed. Testing is typically done in the sleep laboratory, but home testing equipment can distinguish between central and obstructive events. Treatments are limited. Mask-based therapies have been the primary treatment. Oxygen has some data but lacks long-term studies. Neurostimulation of the phrenic nerve is a new technology that has demonstrated improvement. Coordination of care between sleep specialists and cardiologists is important as the field of central sleep apnea continues to develop.

Preface

Sleep and the Heart: What's Next?

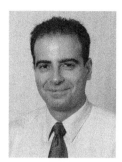

Rami N. Khayat, MD
Editor

The important relationship between cardiovascular disease (CVD) and sleep medicine was recognized in the early years following the emergence of sleep medicine itself as an independent field of Medicine in the 1970s.[1,2] The study of the relationship between sleep and the heart has grown exponentially over the past few decades. Although the areas of interaction between sleep and cardiovascular health are numerous, most of the focus over the past few decades has been on the relationship between sleep-disordered breathing (SDB) and heart failure or other advanced cardiovascular disorders, such as stroke and coronary disease. This was further spurred by the advent and dissemination of highly effective pressure-based devices that address various types of SDB simultaneously.[3] These devices include the various forms of positive airway pressure and the advanced adaptive servo-ventilation technology (ASV).[4,5] The ability to treat all forms of SDB in different populations of patients with one device resulted in less focus on understanding the mechanism of action in different populations such as heart failure patients. Initial, albeit often small, studies consistently showed cardiovascular benefit from treatment of SDB in patients with heart failure and CVD.[6–8] However, when more adequately powered randomized controlled trials were conducted, the results were either neutral or negative. More recently, a trial suggested possible harm of treating central sleep apnea in patients with heart failure and reduced ejection fraction.[9] Another trial showed no effect of treatment of obstructive sleep apnea with continuous positive airway pressure on cardiovascular events in

patients with CVD.[10] These recent p-negative trials showing no benefit from treating SDB in patients with CVD may have stemmed from our inadequate understating of the pathophysiologic relation between SDB and CVD, and from understudy of the effects of positive airway pressure devices. Nevertheless, these trials will unquestionably promulgate critical evaluations of our accepted notions regarding the cardiovascular consequences of SDB. As a result, this field of study is likely to undergo a period of reorganization and consideration of priorities.

On this background, this issue of *Sleep Medicine Clinics* attempts to identify and address this field with a more nuanced view. This issue includes reviews that address the application of current trial findings to clinical practice. In addition, other reviews attempt to address areas in this field that has received less attention in related publications and conferences. The review by Randerath and Herkenrath critically evaluates the current literature on treatment of SDB in patients with CVD, including the recent negative trials, to formulate a nuanced and clinically relevant approach to this important topic.

SDB is associated with increased norepinephrine levels and upregulated sympathetic tone.[11] The consequences of increased sympathetic activation are critical in heart failure patients.[12–14] The consequences of SNA in failing heart include predisposition to ventricular tachyarrhythmia[15] and possibly life-threatening arrhythmia.[16] SDB may therefore represent a critical factor in increasing mortality in HF via arrhythmogenic mechanisms.

Sleep Med Clin 12 (2017) xiii–xiv
http://dx.doi.org/10.1016/j.jsmc.2017.03.002
1556-407X/17/© 2017 Published by Elsevier Inc.

The electrophysiologic underpinnings of this relationship remain unclear and understudied. The review by Oldenburg at al focuses on an important area of interaction between SDB and arrhythmia. In another review, Kahwash presents a clinically generalizable management approach to SDB in patients with CVD.

Other reviews in this issue present novel perspectives on areas that are routinely underrecognized in this field. Dr Jafari discusses the role of SDB in the rehabilitation outcome of patients with CVD. Dr Khan addresses the relation between nonrespiratory sleep disorders and cardiovascular outcomes. This relation can have an impact on the functional outcomes and quality of life in patients with established CVD. Nonrespiratory disorders of sleep are also gaining recognition as a risk factor for the development of CVD in otherwise healthy individuals.

In preparing these reviews, the authors attempted to incorporate the most recent literature in their discussion. These reviews, nevertheless, attempt to formulate and present novel and clinically applicable approaches guided by these recent literature findings. We hope that clinicians can use these reviews in their decision-making and management plans, while still challenging many of the accepted concepts and generating more questions that would advance our field.

Rami N. Khayat, MD
Division of Pulmonary, Allergy, Critical Care, and
Sleep Medicine
Department of Internal Medicine
Davis Heart & Lung Research Institute
The Ohio State University
473 West 12th Avenue, Suite 201
Columbus, OH 43210-1267, USA

E-mail address:
Rami.Khayat@osumc.edu

REFERENCES

1. Tilkian AG, Guilleminault C, Schroeder JS, et al. Sleep-induced apnea syndrome. Prevalence of cardiac arrhythmias and their reversal after tracheostomy. Am J Med 1977;63:348–58.

2. Tilkian AG, Guilleminault C, Schroeder JS, et al. Hemodynamics in sleep-induced apnea. Studies during wakefulness and sleep. Ann Intern Med 1976; 85:714–9.

3. Teschler H, Dohring J, Wang YM, et al. Adaptive pressure support servo-ventilation: a novel treatment for Cheyne-Stokes respiration in heart failure. Am J Respir Crit Care Med 2001;164:614–9.

4. Javaheri S, Brown LK, Randerath WJ. Positive airway pressure therapy with adaptive servoventilation: part 1: operational algorithms. Chest 2014; 146:514–23.

5. Javaheri S, Brown LK, Randerath WJ. Clinical applications of adaptive servoventilation devices: part 2. Chest 2014;146:858–68.

6. Kaneko Y, Floras JS, Usui K, et al. Cardiovascular effects of continuous positive airway pressure in patients with heart failure and obstructive sleep apnea. N Engl J Med 2003;348:1233–41.

7. Duran-Cantolla J, Aizpuru F, Montserrat JM, et al. Continuous positive airway pressure as treatment for systemic hypertension in people with obstructive sleep apnoea: randomised controlled trial. BMJ 2010;341:c5991.

8. Mansfield DR, Gollogly NC, Kaye DM, et al. Controlled trial of continuous positive airway pressure in obstructive sleep apnea and heart failure. Am J Respir Crit Care Med 2004;169:361–6.

9. Cowie MR, Woehrle H, Wegscheider K, et al. Adaptive servo-ventilation for central sleep apnea in systolic heart failure. N Engl J Med 2015;373: 1095–105.

10. McEvoy RD, Antic NA, Heeley E, et al. CPAP for prevention of cardiovascular events in obstructive sleep apnea. N Engl J Med 2016;375:919–31.

11. Somers VK, Dyken ME, Clary MP, et al. Sympathetic neural mechanisms in obstructive sleep apnea. J Clin Invest 1995;96:1897–904.

12. Naughton MT, Benard DC, Liu PP, et al. Effects of nasal CPAP on sympathetic activity in patients with heart failure and central sleep apnea. Am J Respir Crit Care Med 1995;152:473–9.

13. Naughton MT, Liu PP, Bernard DC, et al. Treatment of congestive heart failure and Cheyne-Stokes respiration during sleep by continuous positive airway pressure. Am J Respir Crit Care Med 1995;151: 92–7.

14. Hall AB, Ziadi MC, Leech JA, et al. Effects of short-term continuous positive airway pressure on myocardial sympathetic nerve function and energetics in patients with heart failure and obstructive sleep apnea: a randomized study. Circulation 2014;130:892–901.

15. Javaheri S. Effects of continuous positive airway pressure on sleep apnea and ventricular irritability in patients with heart failure. Circulation 2000;101: 392–7.

16. Bitter T, Westerheide N, Prinz C, et al. Cheyne-Stokes respiration and obstructive sleep apnoea are independent risk factors for malignant ventricular arrhythmias requiring appropriate cardioverter-defibrillator therapies in patients with congestive heart failure. Eur Heart J 2011; 32:61–74.

Sleep Architecture and Blood Pressure

Behrouz Jafari, MD[a,b],*

KEYWORDS

- Sleep physiology • Cardiovascular physiology • Cardiorespiratory coupling • Arousal • REM
- Non-REM

KEY POINTS

- Heart rate and blood pressure have a circadian rhythm characterized by a significant reduction during nighttime hours.
- During non–rapid eye movement sleep, there is an increase in parasympathetic drive and a reduction in cardiac sympathetic activity.
- By contrast, rapid eye movement sleep is a state of autonomic instability, dominated by remarkable fluctuations between parasympathetic and sympathetic influences.
- Any changes in sleep quality, associated with persistence of high sympathetic activity and reduction in physiologic nocturnal blood pressure dipping, results in increased blood pressure during the following days.
- Multiple cardiovascular conditions appear to have sleep-related disturbed autonomic regulation as their basis.

INTRODUCTION

Physiologic regulation during sleep varies with the state of the brain and is influenced by different stages of sleep. On the other hand, control of circulation during sleep requires coordination of the respiratory and the cardiovascular system. All these physiologic systems need to continuously interact with each other and at the same time each one has its own regulatory mechanisms, which adds more complexity to the sleep physiology. In normal circumstances, the heart rate (HR) is constantly being adjusted within each respiratory cycle and depends on the breathing frequency, known as respiratory sinus arrhythmia.[1] To date, little is known about the neural mechanisms of sleep-specific central commands. It is known that different sleep stages modulate regional blood flow at all levels of the nervous system. The strong relation between blood flow and metabolism in the central nervous system indicates that sleep modulates the activity of multiple pathways potentially involved in central autonomic control.[2] As sleep typically involves disengagement from the environment, blood pressure (BP) decreases at night. However, a variety of changes in brain activity during sleep have an effect on physiologic regulation beyond what occurs during wakefulness,[3] so these changes are not just because of disengagement from external environment.

The neural circulatory regulation appears to be coupled with the circadian rhythm; the sleep-wake cycle, including rapid eye movement (REM) and non–rapid eye movement sleep (NREMS) processes, is implicated in long-term BP regulation. The transition from wakefulness to NREMS is characterized by a relative autonomic stability

Disclosure Statement: The author has nothing to disclose.
[a] Section of Pulmonary, Critical Care and Sleep Medicine, School of Medicine, University of California-Irvine, 333 City Boulevard West, Suite 400, Orange, CA 92868-3298, USA; [b] VA Long Beach Healthcare System, 5901 East 7th Street, Long Beach, CA 90822, USA
* VA Long Beach Healthcare System, 5901 East 7th Street, Long Beach, CA 90822.
E-mail address: Jafarib@uci.edu

and increase in parasympathetic drive and a reduction in sympathetic activity. As a consequence, HR, arterial BP, cardiac output, and stroke volume decrease, resulting in an overall decreased cardiac workload. Compared with a subject lying supine during wakefulness,[4–6] BP and cardiac output decrease during sleep. During REM sleep, electroencephalographic (EEG) patterns resemble that of wakefulness, but there is marked muscle atonia and intermittent REM. Not only is the EEG pattern similar to quiet wakefulness but also HR, BP, and sympathetic activity increase to levels that are present during relaxed wakefulness.[4,6,7] This phase is being repeated at 90-minute intervals and exhibits a more irregular pattern, with periodic surges in rather and arterial BP. These changes during REM bring more challenges to homeostatic regulation, especially in cardiovascular or pulmonary diseases. REM sleep also diminishes forebrain influence on brainstem, which has an effect on respiratory compensatory mechanisms that help BP management.

In this article, the author reviews the physiologic changes during different stages of sleep and discusses how these systems interact under normal circumstances.

SLEEP AND CARDIOVASCULAR INTERACTION
Changes in Circulatory Control

Under normal circumstances, HR and BP decrease during nighttime. The decrease in BP is about 10% or greater compared with daytime arterial BP, which is commonly known as "dipping." In addition, supine position and inactivity also contribute to a reduction in the double product noted above.[8]

Previous studies showed that measures of parasympathetic activity, such as RR interval (the time elapsed between 2 successive R waves of the QRS signal on the electrocardiogram), change as early as 2 hours before sleep onset,[9] whereas measures of sympathetic function such as catecholamines and pre-ejection period (the time elapsed between the electrical depolarization of the left ventricle and the beginning of ventricular ejection) decrease with the progression of sleep.[6,9,10]

Awakening has its own fascinating process. It induces a step-by-step activation of the sympathetic and adrenal system, which results in increased HR, BP, and plasma catecholamines. These changes during awakening, of course, will be perpetuated by postural changes and physical activity.[9,11]

On the other hand, the circadian rhythm may also play an important role in cardiovascular activity. Studies investigating the role of circadian rhythm showed subjects who were sleep deprived for 24 hours while in the supine position still had the nocturnal decrease in HR, whereas the decrease in nocturnal BP was blunted.[9,12] These changes as mentioned above suggest that parasympathetic activity (eg, HR) is mostly under circadian influences, whereas sympathetic mechanisms are largely related to the wake-sleep cycle. There is growing evidence showing that nocturnal BP is a key predictor of cardiovascular mortality regardless of the daytime BP levels.[12] Therefore, any changes in sleep can result in nocturnal BP increase and development of hypertension.

Cardiovascular Response During Non-Rapid Eye Movement Sleep

NREMS is characterized by autonomic stability due to a high degree of parasympathetic activity and a decrease in sympathetic tone, which results in a decrease in cardiac workload.[6] It has been shown that during relaxed wakefulness BP decreases progressively, but is interrupted during stage N1 of NREMS.[13] Further reductions in BP after sleep onset have been observed during stage N2[13] and deeper stages of NREMS.[14,15] The lowest levels of arterial BP are reached in stage N3 (formerly known as stages III and IV). This decrease in arterial pressure is primarily related to reduction in HR and sympathetic vasomotor tone.[16] However, the reported differences in BP between the early and late stages of NREMS have often been negligible in human subjects.[6,8,17] During NREMS, arousals increase BP variability,[18,19] which is comparable to average nightly decline in systolic pressure in normotensive individuals.[20] The K-complexes, which are spontaneous or stimulus-evoked phasic bursts activity, are also followed by slight increases in BP during NREMS.[6,14,15] It is of note that, despite these changes, the total variability of BP is less in NREMS than in wakefulness,[8,17] which is an expected event, as the variability of local metabolic needs is decreased, given that behavioral engagement with the environment in NREMS compared with the wakefulness is limited. The decrease in BP during NREMS may also be due to a reduction in HR and, hence, in cardiac output, without significant changes in stroke volume or total peripheral conductance.[21] Change in cardiac output or vascular conductance does not follow the operating logic of the arterial baroreflex during wakefulness. Some studies have shown that during NREMS the arterial baroreflex undergoes either a change in sensitivity or a resetting with respect to wakefulness,[6] and NREMS does not show a substantial increase in baroreflex gain with respect to wakefulness. Therefore, the cardiovascular changes of NREMS can be explained by the baroreflex resetting. Taken together, these findings suggest that the hemodynamic patterns of passing from wakefulness to NREMS involve a resetting of the arterial baroreflex, which originates from centrally driven changes in the autonomic outflow to the heart and vessels. In conclusion, NREMS alters the integration between central and baroreflex drives, which produces the phasic autonomic outflow to the cardiovascular system.

Cardiovascular Response During Rapid Eye Movement Sleep

By contrast, REM is a state of autonomic instability, dominated by significant fluctuations between the parasympathetic and sympathetic nervous system. As a result of cortical desynchronization during REM, the cardiovascular and respiratory system become more unstable. Also, high emotions appear to form a majority of the feelings expressed in dreams, so it would not be surprising that measures of cardiovascular activity mirror this state of heightened emotional arousal. In contrast to NREMS, the BP increases in the form of phasic hypertensive events.[6,8,14,21–23] These changes also result from the phasic neural events like muscle twitches,[24] bursts of REMs,[25,26] and pontogeniculo-occipital waves,[27] which can be seen in REM. When muscle tone is temporarily restored during "REM twitches," there is an abrupt surge in BP.[6] It is plausible that REM, particularly phasic REM sleep, may be a potential trigger for cardiovascular events that are reported to occur more frequently in the early morning hours.[6] Of course, the magnitude of these phasic events may be influenced by synchronization among surges of vasoconstriction in different vascular beds. The relationship between the increases in BP and the phasic changes in HR during REM is still insufficiently clarified. This change in BP can be associated with an increase in HR,[6,8,21,23] although some studies showed no change in HR.[17,22] The inconsistent relations between changes in BP and HR suggest that differences in vascular conductance are involved in determining the hemodynamic pattern of REM. The increased sympathetic traffic to peripheral blood vessels, increased BP, and HR can precede periods of sinus arrests during REM[28,29] due to baroreflex-mediated change[30] and similar bursts of vagal activity.[31]

Several studies have shown that the surge in BP and HR has different time courses during the phasic hypertensive events of REM,[26,32,33] and this confirms that these events are driven by increases in vascular resistance rather than increases in cardiac output.[34] Thus, central autonomic commands that act in parallel on the heart and resistance vessels may explain why the increase in HR is temporally, but not causally, associated with the increase in arterial pressure during REM sleep. The data also indicate that the integration between central and baroreflex drives, which produces the cardiovascular autonomic outflow, differs not only between wakefulness and NREMS but also between the 2 sleep states.[35]

In normal individuals, an increase in HR during REM is associated with an increase in coronary blood flow, corresponding to increases in metabolic demand. However, in patients with severe coronary artery disease, these HR surges coincide with phasic decreases in coronary blood flow, resulting in myocardial ischemia.[36]

On the other hand, during tonic REM, sudden decelerations in heart rhythm can occur that are not associated with any change in HR or BP. As a result, in those with underlying long QT, this can trigger arrhythmias.[31]

Arousals

Arousal, which is associated with sympathetic hyperactivity, results in transient increases in HR and BP.[18,37] Short-term arousal stimuli during sleep, such as those that would elicit K-complexes, are often accompanied by brief bursts of sympathetic vasoconstriction and transient increases in HR and BP.[38] HR has 2 stage responses to arousal: first, tachycardia occurs before the cortical arousal and lasts 4 to 5 seconds, followed by bradycardia. An increase in HR has been shown to happen 10 beats before EEG arousal,[39,40] suggesting that sympathetic activation may have a role in arousal. It also appears that sympathetic hyperactivity remains long after the HR and BP returns to baseline.[41] Above changes are very critical in conditions associated with frequent arousals such as sleep apnea, leading to a sustained effect on the cardiovascular system, causing hypertension, even during the daytime.

In addition, elderly patients, as a result of having less stage N3 and more arousals, are less likely to show the expected nocturnal BP decline. These individuals are at increased risk for left ventricular hypertrophy and other cardiovascular events.[42,43]

Cardiorespiratory Coupling During Sleep

Each physiologic system has its own regulatory mechanisms and constantly interacts with other systems. In normal individuals, there is an uninterrupted intermittent modulation in the HR within each breathing cycle, a mechanism known as respiratory sinus arrhythmia.[1] The other form of cardiorespiratory coordination is called phase synchronization. Cardiorespiratory phase synchronization is a manifestation of coupling between cardiac and respiratory systems complementary to respiratory sinus arrhythmia, which is characterized by heartbeats that occur at specific phases of the respiratory oscillator.[44] Respiration influences the autonomic balance and thus affects heartbeat. The sympathetic predominance during the inspiratory phase causes the heart to accelerate (shorter beat-to-beat intervals), whereas expiration inhibits sympathetic output and augments vagal tone, leading to a reduction in HR (prolonging beat-to-beat intervals). Therefore, abnormalities in breathing may have a direct effect on cardiovascular function. These interactions are most evident in patients with sleep-related breathing disorders, such as obstructive sleep apnea (OSA) and central sleep apnea.

Cardiorespiratory phase synchronization is strongly impacted by different stages of sleep, age, and presence of underlying diseases. The highest synchronization between these 2 systems has been seen in the deepest part of sleep with slow wave.[44] On the other hand, aging is associated with a reduction in synchronization.[44] Thus, they have attenuated HR response to sympathetic stimuli despite increased sympathetic drive. This attenuation in synchronization is partly due to loss of cardiac sensitivity to catecholamines.[45]

Also, this HR variability is significantly disrupted after myocardial infarction.[46] This change in HR variability suggests sympathetic dominance in sleep and loss of sleep-related vagal tone. Whether these findings are true for the postmyocardial infarction population in general and what are their pathophysiological implications remain to be determined.

CLINICAL IMPLICATIONS

Different stages of sleep have important consequences for cardiovascular disease. As an example, sudden changes in the autonomic system may have implications in those with tendency to cardiac arrhythmias, particularly sudden death during sleep.[47] Many cardiovascular diseases show a significant circadian pattern and more frequently during sleep (eg, myocardial infarction, unstable angina, ventricular tachyarrhythmias).[48,49] The physiologic changes during REM sleep may be severely disturbed in the setting of pre-existing coronary artery stenosis, suggesting a mechanism to explain the association between REM sleep and nocturnal cardiac ischemia.[50]

On the other hand, absence of the expected nocturnal BP decline as seen in "non-dippers" like OSA patients,[51,52] or an excessive BP decline during sleep known as "extreme dipping," may both have significant cardiovascular consequences.[53] Patients with "extreme dipping" are at risk of nocturnal hypotension, which leads to cerebral ischemia and lacunar infarcts.[54]

Although the BP decline during sleep is physiologic, it is important that this BP reduction should not be potentiated excessively by iatrogenic interventions such as antihypertensive medication, perhaps administered just before sleep. Further reduction in BP may be especially problematic in patients with impaired regulatory mechanisms (as mentioned above), such as elderly individuals or diabetics with autonomic neuropathy.

SUMMARY

Despite the increase in the understanding of sleep and cardiovascular interaction, there are still many gaps in this knowledge. What it is clear is that different stages of sleep or arousal have a major impact on cardiorespiratory function. Autonomic fluctuations influence different aspects of cardiovascular system, including heart rhythm, BP, coronary and cerebral artery blood flow, and ventilation. Although these surges in sympathetic and parasympathetic activity are well tolerated in normal people, patients with heart disease may be at higher risk for different consequences like arrhythmias, heart attack, or stroke. Investigators are faced with many questions to address in the future, such as the genetic and phenotypic differences between non-dippers and excessive dippers. Therefore, a comprehensive understanding of the physiologic responses to normal sleep at every level is important to better understand the mechanisms and implications of changes in these systems occurring during disordered sleep.

REFERENCES

1. Harper RM, Frysinger RC, Marks JD, et al. Cardiorespiratory control during sleep. Ann N Y Acad Sci 1988;533:368–75.
2. Zoccoli G, Walker AM, Lenzi P, et al. The cerebral circulation during sleep: regulation mechanisms and functional implications. Sleep Med Rev 2002; 6(6):443–55.
3. Parmeggiani PL. Behavioral phenomenology of sleep (somatic and vegetative). Experientia 1980; 36(1):6–11.
4. Hornyak M, Cejnar M, Elam M, et al. Sympathetic muscle nerve activity during sleep in man. Brain 1991;114(Pt 3):1281–95.

5. Mancia G. Autonomic modulation of the cardiovascular system during sleep. N Engl J Med 1993; 328(5):347–9.

6. Somers VK, Dyken ME, Mark AL, et al. Sympathetic-nerve activity during sleep in normal subjects. N Engl J Med 1993;328(5):303–7.

7. Hedner J, Ejnell H, Sellgren J, et al. Is high and fluctuating muscle nerve sympathetic activity in the sleep apnoea syndrome of pathogenetic importance for the development of hypertension? J Hypertens Suppl 1988;6(4):S529–31.

8. Van de Borne P, Nguyen H, Biston P, et al. Effects of wake and sleep stages on the 24-h autonomic control of blood pressure and heart rate in recumbent men. Am J Physiol 1994;266(2 Pt 2):H548–54.

9. Burgess HJ, Trinder J, Kim Y, et al. Sleep and circadian influences on cardiac autonomic nervous system activity. Am J Physiol 1997;273(4 Pt 2):H1761–8.

10. Dodt C, Breckling U, Derad I, et al. Plasma epinephrine and norepinephrine concentrations of healthy humans associated with nighttime sleep and morning arousal. Hypertension 1997;30(1 Pt 1):71–6.

11. Linsell CR, Lightman SL, Mullen PE, et al. Circadian rhythms of epinephrine and norepinephrine in man. J Clin Endocrinol Metab 1985;60(6):1210–5.

12. Kerkhof GA, Van Dongen HP, Bobbert AC. Absence of endogenous circadian rhythmicity in blood pressure? Am J Hypertens 1998;11(3 Pt 1):373–7.

13. Carrington MJ, Barbieri R, Colrain IM, et al. Changes in cardiovascular function during the sleep onset period in young adults. J Appl Physiol 2005;98(2):468–76.

14. Coccagna G, Mantovani M, Brignani F, et al. Laboratory note. Arterial pressure changes during spontaneous sleep in man. Electroencephalogr Clin Neurophysiol 1971;31(3):277–81.

15. Tank J, Diedrich A, Hale N, et al. Relationship between blood pressure, sleep K-complexes, and muscle sympathetic nerve activity in humans. Am J Physiol Regul Integr Comp Physiol 2003;285(1): R208–14.

16. Baccelli G, Guazzi M, Mancia G, et al. Neural and non-neural mechanisms influencing circulation during sleep. Nature 1969;223(5202):184–5.

17. Monti A, Medigue C, Nedelcoux H, et al. Autonomic control of the cardiovascular system during sleep in normal subjects. Eur J Appl Physiol 2002;87(2): 174–81.

18. Davies RJ, Belt PJ, Roberts SJ, et al. Arterial blood pressure responses to graded transient arousal from sleep in normal humans. J Appl Physiol 1993; 74(3):1123–30.

19. Morgan BJ, Crabtree DC, Puleo DS, et al. Neurocirculatory consequences of abrupt change in sleep state in humans. J Appl Physiol 1996;80(5):1627–36.

20. Staessen JA, Bieniaszewski L, O'Brien E, et al. Nocturnal blood pressure fall on ambulatory monitoring in a large international database. The "Ad Hoc" Working Group. Hypertension 1997;29(1 Pt 1):30–9.

21. Khatri IM, Freis ED. Hemodynamic changes during sleep. J Appl Physiol 1967;22(5):867–73.

22. Iellamo F, Placidi F, Marciani MG, et al. Baroreflex buffering of sympathetic activation during sleep: evidence from autonomic assessment of sleep macroarchitecture and microarchitecture. Hypertension 2004;43(4):814–9.

23. Snyder F, Hobson JA, Morrison DF, et al. Changes in respiration, heart rate, and systolic blood pressure in human sleep. J Appl Physiol 1964;19:417–22.

24. Mancia G, Baccelli G, Adams DB, et al. Vasomotor regulation during sleep in the cat. Am J Physiol 1971;220(4):1086–93.

25. Gassel MM, Ghelarducci B, Marchiafava PL, et al. Phasic changes in blood pressure and heart rate during the rapid eye movement episodes of desynchronized sleep in unrestrained cats. Arch Ital Biol 1964;102:530–44.

26. Sei H, Morita Y. Acceleration of EEG theta wave precedes the phasic surge of arterial pressure during REM sleep in the rat. Neuroreport 1996;7(18):3059–62.

27. Sei H, Sakai K, Kanamori N, et al. Long-term variations of arterial blood pressure during sleep in freely moving cats. Physiol Behav 1994;55(4):673–9.

28. Baust W, Bohnert B, Riemann O. The regulation of the heart rate during sleep. Electroencephalogr Clin Neurophysiol 1969;27(6):626.

29. Dickerson LW, Huang AH, Nearing BD, et al. Primary coronary vasodilation associated with pauses in heart rhythm during sleep. Am J Physiol 1993; 264(1 Pt 2):R186–96.

30. Guilleminault C, Pool P, Motta J, et al. Sinus arrest during REM sleep in young adults. N Engl J Med 1984;311(16):1006–10.

31. Verrier RL, Lau TR, Wallooppillai U, et al. Primary vagally mediated decelerations in heart rate during tonic rapid eye movement sleep in cats. Am J Physiol 1998;274(4 Pt 2):R1136–41.

32. Berteotti C, Franzini C, Lenzi P, et al. Surges of arterial pressure during REM sleep in spontaneously hypertensive rats. Sleep 2008;31(1):111–7.

33. Silvani A, Asti V, Bojic T, et al. Sleep-dependent changes in the coupling between heart period and arterial pressure in newborn lambs. Pediatr Res 2005;57(1):108–14.

34. Fewell JE. Influence of sleep on systemic and coronary hemodynamics in lambs. J Dev Physiol 1993; 19(2):71–6.

35. Silvani A. Physiological sleep-dependent changes in arterial blood pressure: central autonomic commands and baroreflex control. Clin Exp Pharmacol Physiol 2008;35(9):987–94.

36. Kirby DA, Verrier RL. Differential effects of sleep stage on coronary hemodynamic function during stenosis. Physiol Behav 1989;45(5):1017–20.

37. Sforza E, Jouny C, Ibanez V. Cardiac activation during arousal in humans: further evidence for hierarchy in the arousal response. Clin Neurophysiol 2000; 111(9):1611–9.

38. Noll G, Elam M, Kunimoto M, et al. Skin sympathetic nerve activity and effector function during sleep in humans. Acta Physiol Scand 1994;151(3):319–29.

39. Takeuchi S, Iwase S, Mano T, et al. Sleep-related changes in human muscle and skin sympathetic nerve activities. J Auton Nerv Syst 1994;47(1–2): 121–9.

40. Bonnet MH, Arand DL. Heart rate variability: sleep stage, time of night, and arousal influences. Electroencephalogr Clin Neurophysiol 1997;102(5):390–6.

41. Lombardi F. Chaos theory, heart rate variability, and arrhythmic mortality. Circulation 2000;101(1):8–10.

42. Verdecchia P, Schillaci G, Gatteschi C, et al. Blunted nocturnal fall in blood pressure in hypertensive women with future cardiovascular morbid events. Circulation 1993;88(3):986–92.

43. Verdecchia P, Schillaci G, Guerrieri M, et al. Circadian blood pressure changes and left ventricular hypertrophy in essential hypertension. Circulation 1990;81(2):528–36.

44. Bartsch RP, Schumann AY, Kantelhardt JW, et al. Phase transitions in physiologic coupling. Proc Natl Acad Sci U S A 2012;109(26):10181–6.

45. Crasset V, Mezzetti S, Antoine M, et al. Effects of aging and cardiac denervation on heart rate variability during sleep. Circulation 2001;103(1):84–8.

46. Vanoli E, Adamson PB, Ba L, et al. Heart rate variability during specific sleep stages. A comparison of healthy subjects with patients after myocardial infarction. Circulation 1995;91(7):1918–22.

47. Schwartz PJ, Priori SG, Spazzolini C, et al. Genotype-phenotype correlation in the long-QT syndrome: gene-specific triggers for life-threatening arrhythmias. Circulation 2001;103(1):89–95.

48. Chasen C, Muller JE. Cardiovascular triggers and morning events. Blood Press Monit 1998;3(1):35–42.

49. Cannon CP, McCabe CH, Stone PH, et al. Circadian variation in the onset of unstable angina and non-Q-wave acute myocardial infarction (the TIMI III Registry and TIMI IIIB). Am J Cardiol 1997;79(3):253–8.

50. Nowlin JB, Troyer WG Jr, Collins WS, et al. The association of nocturnal angina pectoris with dreaming. Ann Intern Med 1965;63(6):1040–6.

51. Somers VK, Dyken ME, Clary MP, et al. Sympathetic neural mechanisms in obstructive sleep apnea. J Clin Invest 1995;96(4):1897–904.

52. Narkiewicz K, Montano N, Cogliati C, et al. Altered cardiovascular variability in obstructive sleep apnea. Circulation 1998;98(11):1071–7.

53. Elliott WJ. Circadian variation in the timing of stroke onset: a meta-analysis. Stroke 1998;29(5):992–6.

54. Kario K, Matsuo T, Kobayashi H, et al. Nocturnal fall of blood pressure and silent cerebrovascular damage in elderly hypertensive patients. Advanced silent cerebrovascular damage in extreme dippers. Hypertension 1996;27(1):130–5.

The Effects of Insomnia and Sleep Loss on Cardiovascular Disease

 CrossMark

Meena S. Khan, MD[a,b],*, Rita Aouad, MD[a]

KEYWORDS

- Short sleep duration • Insomnia • Hypertension • Diabetes • Prediabetes • Cardiovascular disease

KEY POINTS

- Chronic insomnia is a pervasive issue in the general population. It is associated with poor quality of life, increased use of heath care resources, and poor mood.
- Those who are sleep deprived or have insomnia have elevated cortisol levels, increased markers of sympathetic system activity, increased metabolic rate, and endothelial dysfunction; all of which are correlated with increased risk of cardiovascular disease and risk factors.
- Both short sleep duration and insomnia are linked to the development of diabetes and hypertension.
- Insomnia is associated with increased risk of cardiovascular disease and mortality, although not all studies show consistent findings of a positive association.
- Evaluation of sleep health may be an important part of the management of those with cardiovascular disease.

INTRODUCTION

Sleep and its impact on health has been increasingly explored over the past few decades. Sleep loss has negative impacts on quality of life, mood, cognitive function, and health. Insomnia and difficulty sleeping are prevalent issues as well, affecting up to 35% of the population at some point in their lives. Insomnia is linked to poor mood, increased use of health care resources, and decreased quality of life as well as possibly cardiovascular risk factors and disease. Studies have shown increased cortisol levels, decreased immunity, and increased markers of sympathetic activity in sleep-deprived healthy subjects and those with chronic insomnia. The literature also shows that subjective complaints consistent with chronic insomnia and shortened sleep time, both independently and in combination, can be associated with development of diabetes, hypertension, and cardiovascular disease. This article explores the relationship and strength of association between insufficient sleep and insomnia with these health conditions.

SLEEP AND HEALTH

Various sleep disorders, such as obstructive sleep apnea and insomnia, have been associated with a variety of health problems and impaired quality of life. Chronic sleep loss can lead to impaired vigilance and performance, slowing of cognitive processes, depressed mood, and poor attention.[1,2] Sleep quality and duration can effect cellular

Disclosure Statement: The authors have nothing to disclose.
[a] Division of Pulmonary, Critical Care, and Sleep Medicine, Department of Internal Medicine, The Ohio State University, Columbus, OH, USA; [b] Department of Neurology, The Ohio State University, Columbus, OH, USA
* Corresponding author. Division of Pulmonary, Critical Care, and Sleep Medicine, Department of Internal Medicine, The Ohio State University, 201 DHLRI, 473 West 12th Avenue, Columbus, OH 43210.
E-mail address: Meena.Khan@osumc.edu

Sleep Med Clin 12 (2017) 167–177
http://dx.doi.org/10.1016/j.jsmc.2017.01.005
1556-407X/17/© 2017 Elsevier Inc. All rights reserved

immunity and cytokine levels, such that a person's immunity can be impaired with even mild sleep loss.[3,4] Impaired sleep is also linked to changes in metabolism, increased caloric intake, and obesity.[5,6] Short sleep duration is associated with deleterious effects on health, such as increased incidence of all-cause mortality, coronary artery disease, type 2 diabetes mellitus, obesity, and hypertension.[7–11] Short sleep duration has multiple causes, including behavior-induced sleep deprivation, obstructive sleep apnea, shift work syndrome, and insomnia.

Insomnia is a sleep disorder plaguing an estimated 15% of the population[12] and often goes untreated. Chronic insomnia is defined by the *International Classification of Sleep Disorders – Third Edition* (**Box 1**) as a patient, or caregiver, describing difficulty falling asleep, maintaining sleep, waking up earlier than desired, resistance to going to bed on an appropriate schedule, or difficulty sleeping without parent or caregiver intervention, associated with at least 1 symptom that is a consequence of the insomnia, for 3 months or more. The 2005 US National Health and Wellness Survey showed that insomnia is associated with a subjective feeling of decreased quality of life and increased mental health symptoms as well as increased absenteeism from work and decreased work productivity.[13] Insomnia is associated with increased reports of heart disease, high blood pressure, chronic pain, and development of depression and anxiety[14–16] as well as increased use of medical resources and economic burden.[17] Subjective complaints of insomnia and increased sleeping pill use are associated with increased mortality.[18,19] Although the link to mortality has not been demonstrated in all studies,[20–22] this possible association emphasizes the importance of sleep on health.

SLEEP AND ITS EFFECTS ON IMMUNITY AND METABOLIC ACTIVITY

Sleep can influence measures of immunity as well as metabolism and inflammation. There are several possible mechanisms of how insomnia and sleep loss may lead to cardiovascular disease and associated risk factors. Immunity can be divided into adaptive and innate immunity, both of which are regulated by circadian rhythms as well as by sleep. Adaptive immunity refers to immunity that is acquired against a live pathogen to which the organism was previously exposed. Innate immunity refers to defense mechanisms against any foreign body that develop within hours of exposure. The distribution of immune cells is circadian related. Leukocytes, granulocytes, monocytes, and major

---

Box 1
Diagnostic criteria of chronic insomnia

Need A–F to be met

A. The patient reports, or the patient's parent or caregiver observes, 1 or more of the following:

  1. Difficulty initiating sleep

  2. Difficulty maintaining sleep

  3. Waking up earlier than desired

  4. Resistance to going to bed on appropriate schedule

  5. Difficulty sleeping without parent or caregiver intervention

B. The patient reports, or patient's parent or caregiver observes, 1 or more of the following related to the nighttime sleep difficulty:

  1. Fatigue/malaise

  2. Attention, concentration, or memory impairment

  3. Impaired social, family, occupational, or academic performance.

  4. Mood disturbance/irritability

  5. Daytime sleepiness

  6. Behavioral problems

  7. Reduced motivation/energy/initiative

  8. Proneness for errors/accidents

  9. Concern about or dissatisfaction with sleep

C. The reported sleep/wake complaints cannot be explained purely by inadequate opportunity or inadequate circumstances for sleep.

D. The sleep disturbance and associated daytime symptoms occur at least 3 times per week.

E. The sleep disturbance and associated daytime symptoms have been present for at least 3 months.

F. The sleep wake difficulty is not better explained by another sleep disorder.

From American Academy of Sleep Medicine. The International classification of sleep disorders, 3rd edition. Darien (IL): American Academy of Sleep Medicine; 2014; with permission.

---

lymphocytes reach peak levels in the early evening and decline throughout the night.[23] Alternatively, the immune cells responsible for the adaptive immune system are regulated by sleep, during which the levels of interleukin (IL)-2, interferon-∞, and IL-12[24–26] increase. Nocturnal sleep also regulates innate immunity by increasing natural killer cells during sleep and increasing levels the further the night progresses.[27] Sleep loss leads to a decrease in IL-2[23] and chronic insomnia is associated with a decrease in CD3, CD4, and CD8 counts.[28] A loss of natural killer cells and an increase in proinflammatory cytokines, such as IL-6, are also seen during nocturnal sleep.[29] Clinically, sleep loss is associated with decreased immune response to vaccinations and increased susceptibility to infections, such as pneumonia, herpes zoster, and the common cold.[30–34]

The sympathetic nervous system and endocrine system are also affected by sleep. Experimental sleep loss has been demonstrated to lead to alterations in these systems, reflecting a proinflammatory state that can lead to obesity and cardiovascular risk. Sleep fragmentation for 5 months in mice models was shown to cause vascular endothelial dysfunction and increased blood pressure changes.[35] Norepinephrine and epinephrine are normally decreased during sleep, although the degree of change across stages is not definable due to conflicting data.[36–38] Partial sleep deprivation is associated with increased sympathetic activity; a study looking at sleep loss of 3 hours for 1 night only showed increased norepinephrine and epinephrine levels during sleep.[39] Restricting sleep in healthy individuals can increase hunger, impair glucose tolerance, decrease insulin sensitivity, increase cortisol levels, and increase sympathetic system activity.[40–43] Reducing slow wave sleep in particular can result in reduced insulin sensitivity and increased glucose tolerance, even if the total sleep time remains the same.[44] A randomized crossover study by Rao and colleagues[45] compared 5 nights of normal sleep with 5 nights of partial sleep deprivation (4 hours in bed) in 14 healthy subjects and found the partial sleep deprivation group had signs of decreased insulin sensitivity, increased cortisol, and increased catecholamine levels, all of which are indicators of increased stress.[45] The increased hunger, impaired glucose tolerance, and other metabolic changes that occur as a result of sleep restriction may lead to an increased risk of obesity, diabetes, and other cardiovascular risk factors.[43]

The consequences of sleep deprivation to the sympathetic and endocrine systems have been demonstrated in insomnia subjects as well. Chronic insomniacs have higher evening corticotropin and cortisol levels compared with age-matched and body mass index (BMI)–matched healthy controls.[46] Increased arousals during sleep are associated with elevated evening cortisol levels in both chronic insomniacs and age-matched and gender-matched healthy controls.[47] Increased wake time is correlated with increased 24-hour cortisol levels, whereas increased catecholamine levels are associated with increased stage 1 and decreased stage 3 sleep in chronic insomniacs.[48] Insomniacs also have an increased metabolic rate, defined as increased whole body oxygen consumption, compared with age-matched, gender-matched, and weight-matched controls,[49] as well as increased heart rate.[50] These observed metabolic changes may be an underlying mechanism for increased cardiovascular risk factors and disease.

SLEEP LOSS, INSOMNIA, AND DIABETES

Diabetes mellitus is a disease characterized by hyperglycemia that is due to defects in insulin secretion, insulin activity, or both.[51] Chronically elevated blood glucose leads to end organ damage in several organ systems, including the heart and blood vessels, making it a risk factor for cardiovascular disease. Type 2 diabetes mellitus, the most prevalent form of diabetes,[51] is characterized by insulin resistance and inadequate insulin secretion. Glucose intolerance predates diabetes, and if not managed, advances to full-blown type 2 diabetes mellitus. Sleep loss and insomnia are associated with increased prevalence and incidence of both glucose intolerance and type 2 diabetes mellitus. Experimental sleep deprivation on healthy subjects has demonstrated the development of insulin resistance and decreased insulin sensitivity, which are early indicators of developing glucose intolerance and diabetes. Insulin resistance has been induced after just 1 week of partial sleep deprivation in healthy subjects.[52] This has been demonstrated by serum measures of insulin resistance as well as in metabolic markers in the actual adipocyte tissue.[53] Using the hyperinsulinemic-euglycemic clamp, an increase in endogenous glucose production and a decrease in glucose disposal rate, indicating increased insulin resistance, was demonstrated by Donga and colleagues[54] when comparing 1 night of partial sleep deprivation of 4 hours to normal sleep duration in healthy men and women. Even 1 night of partial sleep deprivation can result in a decrease in insulin sensitivity when measured by the homeostasis model assessment (HOMA) index.[55]

The consequences of poor sleep on glucose metabolism have also been demonstrated in clinical studies analyzing the prevalence and incidence of prediabetes and diabetes in those with insufficient or disturbed sleep. Cross-sectional studies reveal an association between decreased sleep time and increased prevalence of diabetes. A cross-sectional analysis of the Sleep Heart

Health Study cohort indicated that short sleep time of less than 6 hours, with or without subjective complaints of insomnia, was significantly associated with the increased prevalence of diabetes or glucose intolerance.[56] Another cross-sectional study by Chao and colleagues[57] found that short sleep duration of less than 6 hours is independently associated with increased prevalence of type 2 diabetes mellitus, even after controlling for other risk factors, such as age, gender, obesity, family history of diabetes, tobacco use, and alcohol consumption. No significant association was found with prediabetes in this study. Prospective studies also support a possible association between short sleep time and the development of new-onset diabetes and prediabetes. A study by Rafalson and colleagues[58] that followed subjects over a 6-year period found a significant association between the development of impaired fasting glucose and short sleep duration of less than 5 hours a night, even after accounting for other confounding factors. Yaggi and colleagues[59] analyzed the Massachusetts Male Aging Study and found a significant association between sleep duration of less than 6 hours a night and the onset of diabetes, independent of other risk factors. A similar study by Beihl and colleagues[60] also revealed a link between the onset of diabetes and average sleep time of 7 hours or less. Large population-based studies, such as the Nurses' Health Study and the Whitehall II study, reinforce this positive association. Published prospective findings from the Nurses' Health Study indicate that subjective reports of sleep duration less than or equal to 5 hours is associated with incident diagnosis of self-reported symptomatic diabetes over 10 years, even after adjusting for age and BMI.[61] Another subjective survey conducted on men in Sweden found those with complaints of short sleep duration and difficulties maintaining sleep had an increased incidence of reporting new-onset diabetes over a 12-year period, even after adjusting for age, hypertension, snoring, BMI, and depression.[62] Similarly, the Whitehall II study cohort conducted over a 5-year period found those with persistent short sleep of less than 5.5 hours a night had increased incidence of type 2 diabetes mellitus even after adjusting for confounding factors.[63] Although this association was weakened when BMI was accounted for, it maintained a trend for a positive association. Although these studies show comparable results of an independent association between short sleep duration and diabetes, the individual study designs vary in their population composition (1 study had an all-male cohort whereas another an all-female cohort) and amount of sleep loss (1

study looked at sleep duration of less than 5 hours, whereas another looked at less than 7 hours). These differences in individual study construct become inconsequential, however, when considering the association between short sleep duration and incident diabetes is retained in large meta-analysis studies. These study results show that sleep duration of less than 6 hours and even 7 hours is associated with an increased risk of incident type 2 diabetes mellitus.[64,65]

Although the results of these studies on sleep duration are compelling, other questions that can be raised, specifically, is if this association is also found in those with insomnia and if these findings are limited to those with behaviorally induced insufficient sleep. Cross-sectional data show that subjective reports of difficulty maintaining sleep and waking up early are associated with clinically identified prediabetes in some but not all studies.[66,67] Chronic self-reported near-nightly sleep disturbance has been shown associated with incidence of diabetes.[67] Hung and colleagues[68] evaluated sleep quality as measured by the Pittsburg Sleep Quality Index (PSQI) versus purely subjective complaints of poor sleep and diabetes and found that both impaired glucose tolerance and diabetes were associated with higher PSQI scores, reflecting poorer sleep quality. This finding remained significant even after adjusting for age, gender, alcohol use, smoking, exercise, BMI, blood pressure, and lipid levels. Likewise, results from prospective studies illustrate that subjective reports of difficulty initiating and maintaining sleep on a chronic basis are associated with incident diabetes. Some studies, however, support sleep initiation as the perpetrator, some support sleep maintenance, and some support both. Nilsson and colleagues[69] published prospective findings indicating subjective reports of difficulty initiating sleep and regular use of hypnotics were associated with incident diabetes, over 12 years, after adjusting for confounding factors. Another survey of Japanese men showed an association between subjective reports of difficulty initiating and maintaining sleep, often or almost every day, and incidence of type 2 diabetes mellitus, after controlling for other risk factors.[70] In Germany, complaints of difficulty maintaining sleep are associated with higher risk of developing type 2 diabetes over 7.5 years, after adjusting for confounding factors.[71] A meta-analysis looking at the longitudinal study data on sleep disturbance and incidence of type 2 diabetes mellitus revealed that difficulty initiating and maintaining sleep was associated with development of type 2 diabetes mellitus,[10] suggesting that both aspects of insomnia are implicated in this risk. Vgontzas and colleagues[72] used polysomnography as an objective measure of sleep duration in combination with subjective insomnia and found that insomnia with an objective sleep duration of less than 5 hours is associated with a 300% higher odds for type 2 diabetes mellitus compared with those who did not have sleep complaints and slept at least 6 hours a night. Furthermore, Vgontzas and colleagues[72] found that neither insomnia alone nor short sleep duration alone without subjective sleep complaints was associated with an increased odds of diabetes. Not only may insomnia be a risk for the development of diabetes but also it may worsen glycemic control in diabetics. Knutson and colleagues[73] used actigraphy and subjective reports to assess the association between insomnia and glycemic control in both diabetics and nondiabetics as part of the Coronary Artery Risk Development in Young Adults study. This study found that sleep fragmentation in diabetics is associated with a 23% higher fasting glucose level, 48% higher fasting insulin level, and 82% higher HOMA. There was no association found between these measured sleep parameters and glucose levels in nondiabetics. The literature mainly supports a positive association between insufficient sleep resulting from insomnia and the prevalence and incidence of type 2 diabetes mellitus; this association may also hold for prediabetes and impaired glycemic control in diabetics. Given the ubiquitous nature of diabetes, and its consequences of end organ damage and cardiovascular disease, screening for sleep disturbances/insufficient sleep should be considered an essential part of the management of type 2 diabetes mellitus.

SLEEP AND HYPERTENSION

Hypertension is a well-known major risk factor for cardiovascular disease. The prevalence of hypertension worldwide ranges from 5% to 71%, with a prevalence of 29% in the United States.[74,75] Early identification and reduction of risk factors are important parts of health maintenance. A potential association of sleep disorders and poor sleep with hypertension is well documented.[76] Home measurements of blood pressure and heart rate are more variable, day to day and morning to evening, in those with insomnia than those without.[77] Normotensive subjects with chronic insomnia have increased nighttime systolic blood pressure (SBP) and blunting of the normal dip in nocturnal blood pressure compared with age-matched and gender-matched controls without insomnia.[78] A meta-analysis looking at cross-sectional and longitudinal study data on sleep

duration found that short sleep duration is associated with an increased risk of hypertension with an odds ratio of 1.21 (95% CI, 1.09–1.34) and relative risk ratio of 1.23 (95% CI, 1.06–1.42), respectively.[79] The Sleep Heart Health Study conducted a cross-sectional analysis of sleep duration (measured by subjective report and polysomnography) and prevalence of hypertension, defined as SBP 140 mm Hg, diastolic blood pressure (DBP) $\geq$90 mm Hg, or use of medication to treat hypertension. Those with a subjective report of less than 7 hours of sleep per night had a higher odds ratio for hypertension.[80] This persisted even after adjustments for age, gender, race, BMI, and apnea–hypopnea index. The presence of insomnia also did not significantly affect this association and the study found that subjects slept less than what they reported when their subjective report was compared with their polysomnography data. A review of cross-sectional studies on insomnia and hypertension reveals conflicting results. A cross-sectional study exploring hypertension (defined as SBP >140 mm Hg, DBP >90 mm Hg, or use of antihypertensive medications) in chronic insomnia for more than a year (reported as difficulty initiating and maintaining early morning awakening or nonrefreshing sleep for at least a year) and normal sleepers (those without any of these sleep complaints) used polysomnography to objectively measure sleep duration, and found those with complaints of insomnia had a significantly increased risk for hypertension, as did those with sleep duration of less than or equal to 5 hours. The association was much stronger for insomnia than short sleep duration and persisted even after adjusting for confounding factors. The risk of hypertension was additive in those with insomnia and short sleep duration with a 500% increased risk of hypertension.[81] In contrast, Vozoris'[82] cross-sectional analysis of the US National Health and Nutrition Examination Survey, a survey that obtains data annually from a nationally representative sample of the population, did not reveal an association between insomnia and hypertension. The study analyzed the association between insomnia, short sleep duration of less than 6 hours, and hypertension and found that subjective insomnia complaints alone did not correlate with presence of hypertension, whereas insomnia with short sleep duration was associated with subjective report of hypertension but not with objective measures of hypertension.[82] Another multiyear cross-sectional analysis of this same cohort by Vozoris[83] investigated whether a correlation exists between the frequency of insomnia symptoms and the presence of hypertension. On initial analysis, results revealed that an increasing frequency of insomnia (measured at 1–15 times in the past 1 month) was correlated with an increased risk of physician diagnosed hypertension and use of anti-hypertensive medications, but the significance was lost after controlling for confounding factors. A similar trend was observed even after short sleep duration of less than 6 hours was accounted for.[83] A cross-sectional analysis by Cheng and colleagues[84] looking at 2 separate time points on the Evolution of Pathways to Insomnia Cohort followed those with hypertension at the first time point and found that neither increased sleep-onset latency nor increased wake time after sleep onset was correlated with presence of hypertension. Those who had increased wake time after sleep onset of greater than 30 minutes, however, had an increased risk for developing hypertension at the 1 year follow-up, even after accounting for age, gender, race, risk for obstructive sleep apnea, sleep duration, and length of insomnia.[84] This association did not hold true for those with an increased sleep onset time of more than 30 minutes.

Longitudinal studies of insomnia and hypertension also have conflicting results. A prospective analysis of a health examination database in Japanese office workers looked at subjective sleep and development of hypertension (defined as SBP $\geq$140 mm Hg and/or DBP $\geq$90 mm Hg or initiating antihypertensive medication) over 4 years. This study found that those reporting always or sometimes having difficulty initiating or maintaining sleep had a higher incidence of hypertension than those without those complaints, even after adjusting for age, BMI, stress, alcohol, and smoking.[85] Another prospective study on insomnia, objective sleep duration, and incidence of hypertension over 7.5 years found that chronic insomnia for more than a year was statistically associated with increased risk of developing hypertension even after controlling for confounding factors. A synergistic effect was observed with short sleep duration of less than 6 hours, and the combination increased the risk of developing hypertension by 4-fold compared with normal sleepers.[86] In contrast, Phillips and Mannino's[87] analysis of a cohort from the Atherosclerosis Risk in Communities study, looking at the development of incident hypertension over 6 years in those with chronic insomnia, found that subjective complaints of insomnia (difficulty falling asleep, staying asleep, and nonrestorative sleep) are not associated with an increased risk of hypertension.[87] Another analysis of the Cardiovascular Health Study cohort looked at several parameters of subjective sleep complaints (difficulty falling asleep, several awakenings a night, and early morning awakenings),

separately and cohesively to examine if an association exists with development of hypertension over a 6-year time frame. This study did not find a significant association between insomnia complaints and the development of hypertension.[88] Some of the discrepancies in results can be attributed to different methods of assessing subjective insomnia complaints, varying durations of what is considered short sleep, and varying longitudinal timelines of symptom logging. A meta-analysis looking at prospective studies on incident hypertension and presence of insomnia symptoms of at least 1 year, found that short sleep duration, complaints of difficulty maintaining sleep, and early morning awakenings, individually and in combination, are associated with an increased risk of developing hypertension.[89] A recent review looking at cross-sectional and longitudinal data concluded that persistent insomnia was associated with increased blood pressure and hypertension risk after controlling for other risk factors in the middle-aged subjects.[90] Overall, the published data on the association of insomnia and hypertension are conflicting, although meta-analysis studies suggest there is a positive association between chronic insomnia and development of hypertension. Before recommendations can be made for sleep screenings as a potential risk modifier for hypertension, more studies are needed to establish a definite association.

SLEEP AND CARDIOVASCULAR DISEASE

Cardiovascular disease is a widespread public health issue in the United States, with an estimated 2200 Americans dying daily from cardiovascular-related events and an estimated 785,000 Americans believed to have a new coronary attack each year.[91] This phenomenon is due to the high prevalence of risk factors, such as 33.5% of adults with hypertension, 20.7% of adults using tobacco, 15% with hyperlipidemia, and 67% of adults classified as overweight, of whom nearly 34% are obese.[91] In addition to these well-known risk factors, subjective complaints of trouble sleeping have been associated with coronary heart disease and incident myocardial infarction, even after excluding obstructive sleep apnea and controlling for other traditional cardiovascular risk factors.[92–94] A large 6-year prospective study of men in the United States revealed an increased risk of mortality after controlling for age, lifestyle, excessive daytime sleepiness, tranquilizer use, and chronic conditions in those with subjective sleep disturbances.[95] In particular, difficulty initiating sleep and nonrestorative sleep had a significantly increased risk of cardiovascular mortality compared with those without such symptoms, and this association remained significant even after excluding patients with cardiovascular disease and depression and controlling for other risk factors.[95] Underlying mechanisms possibly linking these 2 conditions are increased sympathetic activity and vascular endothelial dysfunction, which have been found in chronic insomniacs and sleep-deprived healthy subjects.[35,46–48] Insomnia is also associated with higher nighttime SBP and blunted dipping of nocturnal blood pressure, which could place those patients at risk for cardiovascular disease.[78] Subjective complaints of regular disturbed sleep have been associated with a higher risks of developing hypertension and dyslipidemia, which further elevate risk for cardiovascular disease.[96]

Studies looking at insomnia and sleep duration, and their associations with cardiovascular disease and mortality, have revealed positive associations with various types of sleep complaints. There are also conflicting results, however, with some trends to association but without statistical significance and some negative results. The studies are heterogeneous in their construct, specifically in terms of questions asked to assess sleep quality, varying length of sleep duration, and varying populations studied, which may account for the differences in results. When looking at insomnia, an analysis of the Atherosclerosis Risk in Communities study cohort spanning 6 years found that having a combination of sleep complaints (trouble falling asleep, staying asleep, and awakening unrefreshed) had a slightly increased risk of developing cardiovascular disease.[87] Mallon and colleagues[97] found a significant risk of cardiovascular mortality in men, but not women, with insomnia. They conducted a prospective 12-year study that revealed insomnia (defined as trouble initiating sleep and habitual sleeping pill use) was independently associated with increased all-cause mortality in women but not cardiovascular mortality. In men, however, trouble falling asleep was independently associated with cardiovascular morality.[97] Prospective data from another study with a longer follow-up of 16 years showed that subjective reports of habitual insomnia were independently associated with all-cause mortality and a trend of increased number of cardiovascular events, although this was not statistically significant.[98] A prospective analysis of the Whitehall II cohort, however, looking at sleep in fatal and nonfatal cardiovascular events over a 15-year follow-up period, found that subjectively disturbed sleep had a statistically significant increased hazard ratio of cardiovascular events after adjusting for confounding factors. Sleep duration of less than 6 hours also shows a

significantly increased risk when combined with insomnia but not when looked at alone.[99] Data from the Nurses' Health Study also support a possible link between short sleep duration and cardiovascular disease and found that when subjects were followed for 10 years, sleep duration of less than or equal to 5 hours was associated with fatal and nonfatal coronary artery disease–related events even after adjusting for factors, such as age, BMI, smoking, diabetes, and hypertension.[100] Both the Whitehall II cohort and the Nurses' Health Study support that sleep duration may be associated with cardiovascular disease. The studies looking specifically at insomnia are, however, conflicting. First-time myocardial infarction risk has been correlated to insomnia in 2 studies, although there are some gender differences between male risk and female risk. Laugsand and colleagues[101] found that regular difficulties with initiating sleep, maintaining sleep, and having nonrestorative sleep was associated with a significant risk of having first-time acute myocardial infarction after controlling for confounding factors, such as BMI, cholesterol, blood pressure, and smoking.[101] Women were found to have a slightly higher relative risk compared with men. When looked at individually, each sleep complaint also carried a significant risk, with trouble initiating sleep having the strongest association. Meisinger and colleagues[102] also found that in a 10-year prospective cohort, difficulty maintaining sleep was associated with an increased risk of incident myocardial infarction in women that weakened but still demonstrated a positive association after controlling for confounding factors. This was not found in the male subjects, and this same trend was seen for short sleep duration of less than 6 hours.

The data on insomnia, sleep duration, and fatal/nonfatal cardiovascular events are conflicting. This can be partly attributed to the heterogeneous nature of the studies, as discussed previously. A recent meta-analysis found that symptoms of difficulty initiating sleep and maintaining sleep and early morning awakenings are associated with an increased risk of cardiovascular mortality, with hazard ratios of 1.45, 1.03, and 1.00, respectively,[95] suggesting that poor sleep may be associated with cardiovascular health and should be considered in the management of cardiovascular disease. Depression has also been associated with increased risk of coronary artery disease and myocardial infarction. In some studies, when depression was accounted for, sleep complaints as a risk factor for cardiovascular disease became less significant.[93] Accounting for depression, along with a more uniform approach of quantifying insomnia, would be helpful in future studies to elucidate the independent role that sleep loss may play in cardiovascular health.

SUMMARY

Sleep deprivation and insomnia have a variety of health implications. They affect cognition, mood, and health. Insomnia is a global public health issue that affects more than a quarter of the US population at any point in time and is associated with decreased quality of life and increased economic burden. This article examines the literature on poor sleep and insomnia and their associations with diabetes, hypertension, and cardiovascular disease. Although some studies produced conflicting results, overall the literature supports a possible association that warrants further investigation. Differing study constructs and methods, such as varying methods of quantifying insomnia and inconsistencies, in screening for other confounding sleep disorders, such as obstructive sleep apnea, may explain the conflicting results. Despite these discrepancies, however, there is value in the screening of patients with cardiovascular disease or risk factors for sleep disturbances, especially in regard to improving their health outcomes and quality of life.

REFERENCES

1. Cohen DA, Wang W, Wyatt JK, et al. Uncovering residual effects of chronic sleep loss on human performance. Sci Transl Med 2010;2(14):14ra3.
2. Banks S, Dinges DF. Behavioral and physiological consequences of sleep restriction. J Clin Sleep Med 2007;3(5):519–28.
3. Irwin M. Effects of sleep and sleep loss on immunity and cytokines. Brain Behav Immun 2002; 16(5):503–12.
4. Spiegel K, Sheridan JF, Van Cauter E. Effect of sleep deprivation on response to immunization. JAMA 2002;288(12):1471–2.
5. Broussard JL, Van Cauter E. Disturbances of sleep and circadian rhythms: novel risk factors for obesity. Curr Opin Endocrinol Diabetes Obes 2016;23(5):353–9.
6. Nedeltcheva AV, Kilkus JM, Imperial J, et al. Sleep curtailment is accompanied by increased intake of calories from snacks. Am J Clin Nutr 2009;89(1): 126–33.
7. Cappuccio FP, Stranges S, Kandala NB, et al. Gender-specific associations of short sleep duration with prevalent and incident hypertension: the Whitehall II study. Hypertension 2007;50(4):693–700.
8. Gangwisch JE, Heymsfield SB, Boden-Albala B, et al. Short sleep duration as a risk factor for hypertension: analyses of the first national health and nutrition examination survey. Hypertension 2006;47(5):833–9.
9. Cappuccio FP, D'Elia L, Strazzullo P, et al. Sleep duration and all-cause mortality: a systematic review and meta-analysis of prospective studies. Sleep 2010;33(5):585–92.
10. Cappuccio FP, D'Elia L, Strazzullo P, et al. Quantity and quality of sleep and incidence of type 2 diabetes: a systematic review and meta-analysis. Diabetes Care 2010;33(2):414–20.
11. Tobaldini E, Costantino G, Solbiati M, et al. Sleep, sleep deprivation, autonomic nervous system and cardiovascular diseases. Neurosci Biobehav Rev 2017;74(Pt B):321–9.
12. Chung KF, Yeung WF, Ho FY, et al. Cross-cultural and comparative epidemiology of insomnia: the Diagnostic and statistical manual (DSM), International classification of diseases (ICD) and International classification of sleep disorders (ICSD). Sleep Med 2015;16(4):477–82.
13. Bolge SC, Doan JF, Kannan H, et al. Association of insomnia with quality of life, work productivity, and activity impairment. Qual Life Res 2009;18(4): 415–22.
14. Taylor DJ, Mallory LJ, Lichstein KL, et al. Comorbidity of chronic insomnia with medical problems. Sleep 2007;30(2):213–8.
15. Neckelmann D, Mykletun A, Dahl AA. Chronic insomnia as a risk factor for developing anxiety and depression. Sleep 2007;30(7):873–80.
16. Riemann D, Voderholzer U. Primary insomnia: a risk factor to develop depression? J Affect Disord 2003;76(1–3):255–9.
17. Ozminkowski RJ, Wang S, Walsh JK. The direct and indirect costs of untreated insomnia in adults in the United States. Sleep 2007;30(3):263–73.
18. Pollak CP, Perlick D, Linsner JP, et al. Sleep problems in the community elderly as predictors of death and nursing home placement. J Community Health 1990;15(2):123–35.
19. Kripke DF, Garfinkel L, Wingard DL, et al. Mortality associated with sleep duration and insomnia. Arch Gen Psychiatry 2002;59(2):131–6.
20. Althuis MD, Fredman L, Langenberg PW, et al. The relationship between insomnia and mortality among community-dwelling older women. J Am Geriatr Soc 1998;46(10):1270–3.
21. Foley DJ, Monjan AA, Brown SL, et al. Sleep complaints among elderly persons: an epidemiologic study of three communities. Sleep 1995;18(6): 425–32.
22. Phillips B, Mannino DM. Does insomnia kill? Sleep 2005;28(8):965–71.
23. Born J, Lange T, Hansen K, et al. Effects of sleep and circadian rhythm on human circulating immune cells. J Immunol 1997;158(9):4454–64.

24. Lange T, Dimitrov S, Fehm HL, et al. Shift of mono-cyte function toward cellular immunity during sleep. Arch Intern Med 2006;166(16):1695–700.

25. Lissoni P, Rovelli F, Brivio F, et al. Circadian secretions of IL-2, IL-12, IL-6 and IL-10 in relation to the light/dark rhythm of the pineal hormone melatonin in healthy humans. Nat Immun 1998;16(1):1–5.

26. Petrovsky N, McNair P, Harrison LC. Diurnal rhythms of pro-inflammatory cytokines: regulation by plasma cortisol and therapeutic implications. Cytokine 1998;10(4):307–12.

27. Kronfol Z, Nair M, Zhang Q, et al. Circadian immune measures in healthy volunteers: relationship to hypothalamic-pituitary-adrenal axis hormones and sympathetic neurotransmitters. Psychosom Med 1997;59(1):42–50.

28. Savard J, Laroche L, Simard S, et al. Chronic insomnia and immune functioning. Psychosom Med 2003;65(2):211–21.

29. Irwin MR. Why sleep is important for health: a psychoneuroimmunology perspective. Annu Rev Psychol 2015;66:143–72.

30. Cohen S, Doyle WJ, Alper CM, et al. Sleep habits and susceptibility to the common cold. Arch Intern Med 2009;169(1):62–7.

31. Patel SR, Malhotra A, Gao X, et al. A prospective study of sleep duration and pneumonia risk in women. Sleep 2012;35(1):97–101.

32. Miller GE, Cohen S, Pressman S, et al. Psychological stress and antibody response to influenza vaccination: when is the critical period for stress, and how does it get inside the body? Psychosom Med 2004;66(2):215–23.

33. Prather AA, Hall M, Fury JM, et al. Sleep and antibody response to hepatitis B vaccination. Sleep 2012;35(8):1063–9.

34. Pressman SD, Cohen S, Miller GE, et al. Loneliness, social network size, and immune response to influenza vaccination in college freshmen. Health Psychol 2005;24(3):297–306.

35. Carreras A, Zhang SX, Peris E, et al. Chronic sleep fragmentation induces endothelial dysfunction and structural vascular changes in mice. Sleep 2014; 37(11):1817–24.

36. Somers VK, Dyken ME, Mark AL, et al. Sympathetic-nerve activity during sleep in normal subjects. N Engl J Med 1993;328(5):303–7.

37. Esler M, Jennings G, Lambert G, et al. Overflow of catecholamine neurotransmitters to the circulation: source, fate, and functions. Physiol Rev 1990; 70(4):963–85.

38. Wallin BG. Relationship between sympathetic nerve traffic and plasma concentrations of noradrenaline in man. Pharmacol Toxicol 1988; 63(Suppl 1):9–11.

39. Irwin M, Thompson J, Miller C, et al. Effects of sleep and sleep deprivation on catecholamine and interleukin-2 levels in humans: clinical implications. J Clin Endocrinol Metab 1999;84(6):1979–85.

40. Spiegel K, Leproult R, Van Cauter E. Impact of sleep debt on metabolic and endocrine function. Lancet 1999;354(9188):1435–9.

41. Leproult R, Copinschi G, Buxton O, et al. Sleep loss results in an elevation of cortisol levels the next evening. Sleep 1997;20(10):865–70.

42. Stamatakis KA, Punjabi NM. Effects of sleep fragmentation on glucose metabolism in normal subjects. Chest 2010;137(1):95–101.

43. Van Cauter E, Holmback U, Knutson K, et al. Impact of sleep and sleep loss on neuroendocrine and metabolic function. Horm Res 2007;67(Suppl 1):2–9.

44. Tasali E, Leproult R, Ehrmann DA, et al. Slow-wave sleep and the risk of type 2 diabetes in humans. Proc Natl Acad Sci U S A 2008;105(3):1044–9.

45. Rao MN, Neylan TC, Grunfeld C, et al. Subchronic sleep restriction causes tissue-specific insulin resistance. J Clin Endocrinol Metab 2015;100(4): 1664–71.

46. Vgontzas AN, Bixler EO, Lin HM, et al. Chronic insomnia is associated with nyctohemeral activation of the hypothalamic-pituitary-adrenal axis: clinical implications. J Clin Endocrinol Metab 2001; 86(8):3787–94.

47. Rodenbeck A, Huether G, Rüther E, et al. Interactions between evening and nocturnal cortisol secretion and sleep parameters in patients with severe chronic primary insomnia. Neurosci Lett 2002; 324(2):159–63.

48. Vgontzas AN, Tsigos C, Bixler EO, et al. Chronic insomnia and activity of the stress system: a preliminary study. J Psychosom Res 1998;45(1):21–31.

49. Bonnet MH, Arand DL. 24-Hour metabolic rate in insomniacs and matched normal sleepers. Sleep 1995;18(7):581–8.

50. Bonnet MH, Arand DL. Heart rate variability in insomniacs and matched normal sleepers. Psychosom Med 1998;60(5):610–5.

51. Report of the expert committee on the diagnosis and classification of diabetes mellitus. Diabetes Care 1997;20(7):1183–97.

52. Buxton OM, Pavlova M, Reid EW, et al. Sleep restriction for 1 week reduces insulin sensitivity in healthy men. Diabetes 2010;59(9):2126–33.

53. Broussard JL, Ehrmann DA, Van Cauter E, et al. Impaired insulin signaling in human adipocytes after experimental sleep restriction: a randomized, crossover study. Ann Intern Med 2012;157(8): 549–57.

54. Donga E, van Dijk M, van Dijk JG, et al. A single night of partial sleep deprivation induces insulin resistance in multiple metabolic pathways in healthy subjects. J Clin Endocrinol Metab 2010; 95(6):2963–8.

55. Cedernaes J, Osler ME, Voisin S, et al. Acute sleep loss induces tissue-specific epigenetic and transcriptional alterations to circadian clock genes in men. J Clin Endocrinol Metab 2015;100(9):E1255–61.

56. Gottlieb DJ, Punjabi NM, Newman AB, et al. Association of sleep time with diabetes mellitus and impaired glucose tolerance. Arch Intern Med 2005;165(8):863–7.

57. Chao CY, Wu JS, Yang YC, et al. Sleep duration is a potential risk factor for newly diagnosed type 2 diabetes mellitus. Metabolism 2011;60(6):799–804.

58. Rafalson L, Donahue RP, Stranges S, et al. Short sleep duration is associated with the development of impaired fasting glucose: the Western New York health study. Ann Epidemiol 2010;20(12):883–9.

59. Yaggi HK, Araujo AB, McKinlay JB. Sleep duration as a risk factor for the development of type 2 diabetes. Diabetes Care 2006;29(3):657–61.

60. Beihl DA, Liese AD, Haffner SM. Sleep duration as a risk factor for incident type 2 diabetes in a multi-ethnic cohort. Ann Epidemiol 2009;19(5):351–7.

61. Ayas NT, White DP, Al-Delaimy WK, et al. A prospective study of self-reported sleep duration and incident diabetes in women. Diabetes Care 2003;26(2):380–4.

62. Mallon L, Broman JE, Hetta J. High incidence of diabetes in men with sleep complaints or short sleep duration: a 12-year follow-up study of a middle-aged population. Diabetes Care 2005; 28(11):2762–7.

63. Ferrie JE, Kivimäki M, Akbaraly TN, et al. Change in sleep duration and type 2 diabetes: the Whitehall II study. Diabetes Care 2015;38(8):1467–72.

64. Holliday EG, Magee CA, Kritharides L, et al. Short sleep duration is associated with risk of future diabetes but not cardiovascular disease: a prospective study and meta-analysis. PLoS One 2013; 8(11):e82305.

65. Shan Z, Ma H, Xie M, et al. Sleep duration and risk of type 2 diabetes: a meta-analysis of prospective studies. Diabetes Care 2015;38(3):529–37.

66. Engeda J, Mezuk B, Ratliff S, et al. Association between duration and quality of sleep and the risk of pre-diabetes: evidence from NHANES. Diabet Med 2013;30(6):676–80.

67. Kowall B, Lehnich AT, Strucksberg KH, et al. Associations among sleep disturbances, nocturnal sleep duration, daytime napping, and incident pre-diabetes and type 2 diabetes: the Heinz Nixdorf Recall Study. Sleep Med 2016;21:35–41.

68. Hung H, Yang Y, Ou H, et al. The association between impaired glucose tolerance and self-reported sleep quality in a chinese population. Can J Diabetes 2012;36:95–9.

69. Nilsson PM, Rööst M, Engström G, et al. Incidence of diabetes in middle-aged men is related to sleep disturbances. Diabetes Care 2004;27(10):2464–9.

70. Kawakami N, Takatsuka N, Shimizu H. Sleep disturbance and onset of type 2 diabetes. Diabetes Care 2004;27(1):282–3.

71. Meisinger C, Heier M, Loewel H, et al, MONICA/KORA Augsburg Cohort Study. Sleep disturbance as a predictor of type 2 diabetes mellitus in men and women from the general population. Diabetologia 2005;48(2):235–41.

72. Vgontzas AN, Liao D, Pejovic S, et al. Insomnia with objective short sleep duration is associated with type 2 diabetes: a population-based study. Diabetes Care 2009;32(11):1980–5.

73. Knutson KL, Van Cauter E, Zee P, et al. Cross-sectional associations between measures of sleep and markers of glucose metabolism among subjects with and without diabetes: the Coronary Artery Risk Development in Young Adults (CARDIA) Sleep Study. Diabetes Care 2011;34(5):1171–6.

74. Kearney PM, Whelton M, Reynolds K, et al. Worldwide prevalence of hypertension: a systematic review. J Hypertens 2004;22(1):11–9.

75. Ong KL, Cheung BM, Man YB, et al. Prevalence, awareness, treatment, and control of hypertension among United States adults 1999-2004. Hypertension 2007;49(1):69–75.

76. Bansil P, Kuklina EV, Merritt RK, et al. Associations between sleep disorders, sleep duration, quality of sleep, and hypertension: results from the National Health and Nutrition Examination Survey, 2005 to 2008. J Clin Hypertens (Greenwich) 2011;13(10):739–43.

77. Johansson JK, Kronholm E, Jula AM. Variability in home-measured blood pressure and heart rate: associations with self-reported insomnia and sleep duration. J Hypertens 2011;29(10):1897–905.

78. Lanfranchi PA, Pennestri MH, Fradette L, et al. Nighttime blood pressure in normotensive subjects with chronic insomnia: implications for cardiovascular risk. Sleep 2009;32(6):760–6.

79. Guo X, Zheng L, Wang J, et al. Epidemiological evidence for the link between sleep duration and high blood pressure: a systematic review and meta-analysis. Sleep Med 2013;14(4):324–32.

80. Gottlieb DJ, Redline S, Nieto FJ, et al. Association of usual sleep duration with hypertension: the sleep heart health study. Sleep 2006;29(8):1009–14.

81. Vgontzas AN, Liao D, Bixler EO, et al. Insomnia with objective short sleep duration is associated with a high risk for hypertension. Sleep 2009; 32(4):491–7.

82. Vozoris NT. The relationship between insomnia symptoms and hypertension using United States population-level data. J Hypertens 2013;31(4):663–71.

83. Vozoris NT. Insomnia symptom frequency and hypertension risk: a population-based study. J Clin Psychiatry 2014;75(6):616–23.

84. Cheng P, Pillai V, Mengel H, et al. Sleep maintenance difficulties in insomnia are associated with increased incidence of hypertension. Sleep Health 2015;1:50–4.

85. Suka M, Yoshida K, Sugimori H. Persistent insomnia is a predictor of hypertension in Japanese male workers. J Occup Health 2003;45(6):344–50.

86. Fernandez-Mendoza J, Vgontzas AN, Liao D, et al. Insomnia with objective short sleep duration and incident hypertension: the penn state cohort. Hypertension 2012;60(4):929–35.

87. Phillips B, Mannino DM. Do insomnia complaints cause hypertension or cardiovascular disease? J Clin Sleep Med 2007;3(5):489–94.

88. Phillips B, Bůzková P, Enright P, et al, Cardiovascular Health Study Research Group. Insomnia did not predict incident hypertension in older adults in the cardiovascular health study. Sleep 2009;32(1):65–72.

89. Meng L, Zheng Y, Hui R. The relationship of sleep duration and insomnia to risk of hypertension incidence: a meta-analysis of prospective cohort studies. Hypertens Res 2013;36(11):985–95.

90. Palagini L, Bruno RM, Gemignani A, et al. Sleep loss and hypertension: a systematic review. Curr Pharm Des 2013;19(13):2409–19.

91. Roger VL, Go AS, Lloyd-Jones DM, et al. Heart disease and stroke statistics–2012 update: a report from the American Heart Association. Circulation 2012;125(1):e2–220.

92. Schwartz S, McDowell Anderson W, Cole SR, et al. Insomnia and heart disease: a review of epidemiologic studies. J Psychosom Res 1999;47(4):313–33.

93. Schwartz SW, Cornoni-Huntley J, Cole SR, et al. Are sleep complaints an independent risk factor for myocardial infarction? Ann Epidemiol 1998; 8(6):384–92.

94. Eaker ED, Pinsky J, Castelli WP. Myocardial infarction and coronary death among women: psychosocial predictors from a 20-year follow-up of women in the Framingham Study. Am J Epidemiol 1992; 135(8):854–64.

95. Li Y, Zhang X, Winkelman JW, et al. Association between insomnia symptoms and mortality: a prospective study of U.S. men. Circulation 2014; 129(7):737–46.

96. Clark AJ, Salo P, Lange T, et al. Onset of impaired sleep and cardiovascular disease risk factors: a longitudinal study. Sleep 2016;39(9):1709–18.

97. Mallon L, Broman JE, Hetta J. Sleep complaints predict coronary artery disease mortality in males: a 12-year follow-up study of a middle-aged Swedish population. J Intern Med 2002;251(3):207–16.

98. Chien KL, Chen PC, Hsu HC, et al. Habitual sleep duration and insomnia and the risk of cardiovascular events and all-cause death: report from a community-based cohort. Sleep 2010;33(2):177–84.

99. Chandola T, Ferrie JE, Perski A, et al. The effect of short sleep duration on coronary heart disease risk is greatest among those with sleep disturbance: a prospective study from the Whitehall II cohort. Sleep 2010;33(6):739–44.

100. Ayas NT, White DP, Manson JE, et al. A prospective study of sleep duration and coronary heart disease in women. Arch Intern Med 2003;163(2):205–9.

101. Laugsand LE, Vatten LJ, Platou C, et al. Insomnia and the risk of acute myocardial infarction: a population study. Circulation 2011;124(19):2073–81.

102. Meisinger C, Heier M, Löwel H, et al. Sleep duration and sleep complaints and risk of myocardial infarction in middle-aged men and women from the general population: the MONICA/KORA Augsburg cohort study. Sleep 2007;30(9):1121–7.

Sleep and the Cardiovascular System in Children

Grace R. Paul, MD*, Swaroop Pinto, MD

KEYWORDS

• Sleep • Children • Cardiovascular • Congenital

KEY POINTS

- Cardiovascular (CV) physiology and pathophysiology differ in children compared with adults.
- Obstructive sleep apnea (OSA) and central sleep apnea (CSA) occur in children due to diverse and multifactorial causes.
- Congenital heart disease (CHD), craniofacial anomalies, clinical syndromes, and the related sleep and CV morbidity are unique to the pediatric age group.

INTRODUCTION

Current subspecialty pediatric practice provides comprehensive medical care for a wide range of ages, from premature infants to children, and often includes adults with complex medical and surgical issues that warrant multidisciplinary care. Normal physiologic variations involving different body systems occur during in sleep and these vary with age, stage of sleep, and underlying health conditions. The practice of pediatric sleep medicine is exciting due to the broad changes in cardiopulmonary physiology seen with normal growth and maturation and the plethora of congenital or acquired medical and surgical pathologies affecting this population. Sleep-related breathing disorders in children occur along a spectrum of severity, ranging from mild snoring to severe obstructive apnea, central apnea, and nocturnal hypoventilation. There is limited information available on the bidirectional effect of sleep-disordered breathing (SDB) causing CV morbidity and vice versa, especially in predisposed populations. This article is a concise review of the CV physiology and pathophysiology in children during SDB contributing to CV morbidity, congenital and acquired CV pathology resulting in SDB, and the relationship between SDB and CV morbidity in different clinical syndromes and systemic diseases in the expanded pediatric population.

PHYSIOLOGY AND PATHOPHYSIOLOGY
Cardiovascular Physiology of Sleep in Children

With normal maturation of the neonate into childhood, changes in CV function during sleep reflect maturation of the autonomic nervous system (ANS), with higher parasympathetic control observed with increasing age.[1] An important indicator of ANS activity is beat-to-beat heart rate variability (HRV), and in healthy infants and children, age and sleep stage influence short-term HRV.[2]

Heart rate (HR) and blood pressure (BP) are lower during non–rapid eye movement (NREM) sleep than during wakefulness throughout maturation from the neonatal period to childhood. During transition from quiet wake to quiet sleep stage, HR decreases by 4 beats per minute to 8 beats per minute and BP decreases by approximately 14 mm Hg[3] along with a reduction in cardiac output. During tonic rapid eye movement (REM) state, however, an 8% drop in HR along with a simultaneous drop in BP

Disclosure Statement: The authors have nothing to disclose.
Division of Pulmonary and Sleep Medicine, Nationwide Children's Hospital, The Ohio State University, 700 Children's Drive, Columbus, OH 43205, USA
* Corresponding author.
E-mail address: Grace.Paul@nationwidechildrens.org

sleep.theclinics.com

(up to 25 mm Hg) and a significant reduction in cardiac output (up to 9% drop compared with QW) has been observed.[4,5] HRV is also higher in REM sleep than in NREM sleep, especially during phasic REM sleep. Cutaneous vasoconstriction is noted briefly during REM sleep, along with regional vasoconstriction to specific organ systems.

Pathophysiology

A diminished HR variability with respiration during specific sleep stages has been described in infants with underlying medical or surgical disease, in infants at risk for sudden infant death syndrome (SIDS) or those who later succumbed to SIDS, and in those with hypoventilation syndromes.[6] Autonomic modulation shifts toward parasympathetic activity from wake to NREM and reverses to less parasympathetic modulation during REM sleep in normal children. With moderate SDB, however, autonomic modulation is impaired. This leads to higher arrhythmia vulnerability, especially during REM sleep,[7] although the frequency of nocturnal arrhythmias is less common in children compared with adults with SDB.[8] Children with more disrupted sleep (increased activity, wake after sleep onset, and long wake episodes) had lower respiratory sinus arrhythmia at baseline and reactivity, suggesting increased ANS arousal, which interferes with sleep.[9]

Sleep duration inversely predicts cardiometabolic risk in obese adolescents, even when controlling for physical activity, anthropometry, and adiposity. Long sleep duration has been significantly associated with lower ambulatory systolic and diastolic BP.[10,11] In a cross-sectional study involving more than 300 healthy prepubertal children, however, sleep regularity was more prominently associated with both metabolic regulation (insulin resistance) and inflammation (high-sensitivity C-reactive protein) than sleep duration.[12] The CV pathophysiology of OSA and CSA is discussed.

Although cardiac variations during sleep in newborns, infants, and children are complex in a medically susceptible child, these variations are of clinical significance, especially during phasic excitatory stages of sleep.

SLEEP-DISORDERED BREATHING AND CARDIOVASCULAR DISEASE IN CHILDREN
Obstructive Sleep Apnea

OSA is secondary to intermittent upper airway obstruction (UAO) during sleep, with increased work of breathing, worsened negative intrathoracic pressures, frequent arousals, sleep disruption, and disturbances in blood gas exchange. Long-standing UAO results in CV complications, such as endothelial dysfunction, chronic systemic inflammation via oxidative stress, and increased sympathetic tone resulting in BP abnormalities and CV structural modifications.[13] In healthy individuals, sympathetic output increases in REM sleep and during arousals,[14] with stimulation of chemoreceptors by hypoxia and hypercapnia also increasing sympathetic activity. In patients with OSA, abnormal gas exchanges and arousals augment the sympathetic tone even more along with surges in certain catecholamines,[15,16] which result in vasoconstriction and further elevations in BP.

Few data are available regarding CV morbidity in children with OSA syndrome. In children, exaggerated sympathetic responses and increased HR fluctuations were observed in those with OSA compared with controls[17,18] and treatment of OSA has shown reduction in both sympathetic tone and plasma and urine levels of catecholamines.[19,20]

In small cohort studies of children with snoring and OSA, investigators have reported increased diastolic BP and higher awake BP and systolic BP during REM sleep.[21,22] Pediatric studies with 24-hour ambulatory BP monitoring showed increased BP variability and decreased nocturnal BP dipping.[23,24] In a meta-analysis of pediatric studies, even though not statistically significant, it was observed that during wakefulness, moderate to severe OSA syndrome was associated with an 87% and 121% higher risk for increased systolic and diastolic BP, compared with mild or no OSA, and during sleep, the random effects odds ratio for elevated SBP was 1.2 (95% CI, 0.29–5.02) and fixed effects OR for elevated diastolic BP was 2.23 (95% CI, 0.61–8.16).[25] In summary, the trend is that higher systemic BP (especially the diastolic BP) is observed with greater severity of OSA in children.

Intermittent nocturnal hypoxemia increases oxidative stress and production of leukocyte adherence molecules, which may result in endothelial dysfunction and vascular injury. Chronic hypoxemia, increased sympathetic tone, and exaggerated negative intrathoracic pressures during inspiration against an obstructed airway are important OSA-related consequences affecting preload and afterload on the cardiac ventricles.[13] Chronic mechanical strain to the cardiac ventricles, with reductions in the right ventricular (RV) and left ventricular (LV) stroke volumes due to episodic surges in afterload after fluctuations in the pulmonary and systemic arterial pressures are seen with obstructive events.[26,27] As discussed previously, OSA is associated with LV dysfunction along with RV changes. Amin and colleagues[28] reported that children with higher apnea–hypopnea index had higher risk for increased RV end-diastolic volume and LV mass index and noted a negative correlation between OSA severity and LV diastolic function. In children, brain natriuretic peptide is a good measure of cardiac strain, with correlation between increases in BNP levels and severity of UAO in children reported.[29] Reduction in RV ejection fraction and RV dilatation were noted in children with adenotonsillar hypertrophy, with resolution after surgery.[30,31]

Proinflammatory markers have been implicated in the pathogenesis of OSA. In a randomized prospective multicenter study, plasma samples were assayed for multiple inflammatory markers in healthy obese Spanish children ages 4 years to 15 years. Of the 75 children who had OSA, monocyte chemoattractant protein-1 (MCP-1) and plasminogen activator inhibitor-1 (PAI-1) levels were significantly higher, interleukin-6 (IL-6) concentrations was higher in moderate-severe OSA ($P<.01$), and MCP-1 levels were associated with more prolonged nocturnal hypercapnia ($P<.001$)[32] compared with children without OSA.

Significant reductions in the proinflammatory markers, especially IL-6, IL-18, PAI-1, MCP-1, and matrix metalloproteinase-9, and increases in adropin and osteocrin plasma concentrations occur after adenotonsillectomy for OSA, reflecting the reversibility of the inflammatory activity after OSA treatment.[33] Plasma C-reactive protein is being evaluated as a marker for chronic systemic inflammation in children with OSA, but even though it correlated with adiposity, C-reactive protein levels did not consistently correlate with elevations in AHI.

Recent studies have shown the disturbances in gut microbiome (which is a major homeostatic regulator) by obesity and OSA may lead to increased translocation of bacterial lipopolysaccharides across the gut epithelium into the systemic circulation, leading to metabolic dysfunction.[34–36]

Therefore, similar to obesity, OSA is sometimes viewed as a chronic low-grade inflammatory disease due to its role in the initiation and propagation of localized and systemic inflammatory processes.[37]

In summary, chronic sympathetic overtone and oxidative stress result in BP elevation, insulin resistance, chronic systemic inflammation, endothelial dysfunction, decreased arterial distensibility, and development of atherosclerosis, resulting in significant CV morbidity even in children.[13]

Central Sleep Apnea

CSA in children is a common physiologic phenomenon during sleep. CSA is defined as the absence of chest and abdominal movement associated with a cessation of airflow for more than 20 seconds or lasting more than 2 baseline respiratory cycles if it associated with an arousal an awakening or an oxygen desaturation of at least 3%.[38] It is considered pathologic if the central apnea index is more than 5/h.[39–41]

CSA like OSA is associated with fragmented sleep and excessive daytime sleepiness, but unlike OSA, which results in CV morbidity, CSA often occurs secondary to CV disease.[42,43] There are several manifestations of CSA in children, which vary with age, and there is considerable overlap in the pathogenesis and pathophysiology of OSA and CSA.

Pathophysiology

Unstable ventilatory drive during sleep has been implicated in the pathogenesis of CSA. Central chemoreceptors in the medulla respond to small variations in $Paco_2$ to regulate normal gas exchange and to minimize acid-base changes and peripheral chemoreceptors in the carotid bodies respond to Pao_2 to a larger extent than $Paco_2$. The variability in ventilation leading to unstable breathing can be explained by the loop gain concept.[44–47] Individuals with highly sensitive chemoresponses have increased ventilation for a given increase in $Paco_2$ compared with individuals with low chemosensitivity.[47] Hyperventilation continues until it results in reduction in Pco_2 to below eucapnic level, which is detected at the chemoreceptors, leading to hypoventilation and potential apnea.[46,48,49]

Loop gain is directly proportional to ventilatory sensitivity to hypoxia and hypercapnia; differences between inspired and arterial partial pressures for either O_2 or CO_2 and circulation time between the lung and chemoreceptors. Loop gain is inversely proportional to lung volume.

Cheyne-Stokes respiration is an example of high loop gain. The ventilator response is out of proportion to the change in blood gases and is exacerbated by concomitant congestive heart failure,[50] which causes delayed circulatory times between the lung and chemoreceptors.[51] Periodic breathing (PB) is a similar pattern of respiration often seen in otherwise normal patients between 2 weeks and 6 months of age.[52] The cause of PB is uncertain but may be related to maturation of receptors. PB may also be seen, however, in infants who are hypoxemic. In these cases, infants may have combination of increased chemosensitivity, alterations in arterial O_2 or CO_2, delayed signal transmission between the lung and chemoreceptors, and low lung volumes. These conditions can increase loop gain, resulting in an exacerbated ventilatory response. In infants who are hypoxemic and eucapnic, administration of supplemental oxygen abolishes the PB, suggesting that the carotid body is a primary component responsible to PB.[52,53]

The pathophysiology of CSA is related to changes in stage of sleep with transition from wakefulness to sleep inherently unstable. With sleep onset, there is decreased in upper airway tone leading to increase in upper airway resistance. Change in ventilation due to arousal also contributes to the development of CSA; therefore, OSAs or increased arousals are a risk for CSA.[43,48]

CSA can be isolated CSA (eucapnic or hypocapnic) or associated with hypoventilation (hypercapnia), which can be further divided into primary or secondary. Primary CSA with hypoventilation is seen in congenital central hypoventilation syndrome (CCHS) and secondary CSA with hypoventilation is seen in brainstem lesions, Arnold-Chiari malformations, Joubert syndrome, Prader-Willi syndrome, apnea of prematurity, and obesity.[54–56]

The most common manifestations of CSA in newborns is apnea of prematurity, which is explained by immaturity of the central nervous system leading to poor ventilator responses and causing unstable ventilation leading to CSA. Peak incidence occurs between 47 weeks' and 66 weeks' gestational age, is generally treated with respiratory stimulants like caffeine, and in rare instances may require noninvasive ventilation.[53,57]

Sudden Infant Death Syndrome

According to the Centers for Disease Control and Prevention, SIDS is the sudden death of an infant less than 1 year old that cannot be explained after a thorough investigation, including a complete autopsy, examination of the death scene, and a review of the medical history. SIDS is the leading cause of death for infants ages 1 to 12 months. In a recent prospective, population-based study done in Australia and New Zealand, 49 cases of sudden death were identified in children between 1 year and 5 years of age, and of those deaths 76% were unexplained, 70% occurred in boys, and 91% occurred during sleep ($P<.001$).[58] Clinical screening of these families revealed inherited arrhythmogenic diseases (such as the long QT syndrome, polymorphic ventricular tachycardia, short QT syndrome, and primary conduction disease) and inherited cardiomyopathies (arrhythmogenic RV cardiomyopathy [CM], dilated CM, LV noncompaction, and so forth). Death during sleep may be due to bursts of vagal and sympathetic activity during REM sleep, leading to sympathetically triggered arrhythmias. Vestibular and cerebellar

input to BP regulation varies with age and this age dependency of baroreflex responses plays an important role in some SIDS victims, because they seem to succumb to a drop in BP and HR rather than respiratory failure.[59] Altered vagal reactivity, especially during stress or disease, may provide insight into neuronal disruptions predicting sleep problems, especially considering the increased vulnerability of preterm infants to SIDS.[60]

The interaction between genotype, environment, and the SIDS phenotype is being studied to understand the pathogenesis of SIDS. For example, a mutation in the cardiac sodium channel gene SCN5A, which is associated with altered sodium current, results in action potential prolongation and afterdepolarizations, leading to prolonged QT interval and arrhythmia, eventuating in the clinical phenotype of SIDS.[61] Arrhythmias related and unrelated to ion channelopathies within the cardiac muscle have also been implicated in SIDS.

Congenital Central Hypoventilation Syndrome

CCHS is a rare disorder of respiratory and autonomic regulation, usually presenting in newborns and rarely in older children and adults. Hypoventilation occurs either only during sleep or while awake and sleep, along with ANS dysregulation. PHOX2B gene mutations have been associated with CCHS.

Cardiac abnormalities associated with CCHS include decreased HRV, attenuated HR response to exercise, attenuation of normal sleep-related decrement in BP, and absence of standing-related BP overshoot with potential reduced cerebral regional blood flow.[62]

Children with CCHS are at higher risk for prolonged sinus pauses and asystole, which may need cardiac pacing[63] and, therefore, the current recommended evaluation for CCHS includes 72-hour Holter monitor recording to assess for abrupt, prolonged asystoles, echocardiogram to evaluate for RV hypertrophy and cor pulmonale, and comprehensive autonomic testing of all organ systems regulated by the ANS.

SLEEP MANIFESTATIONS OF CARDIOVASCULAR DISEASE
Congenital Heart Disease

SDB has been often observed in infants with CHD and statistically significant differences in AHI, oxygen nadir, and percentage of total sleep time (TST) with oxygen saturation less than 90% have been observed[64,65] compared with infants without CHD. In 1 study, the median AHIs were 2.5, 2.4, and 0.7 (P = .013) and the O_2 nadirs were 79%, 73%, and 90% ($P<.001$) in the acyanotic, cyanotic CHD infants, and controls, respectively.[64]

Similarly, in a study by Hiatt and colleagues,[65] 19 infants had CHD and 11 were controls. Significant differences were noted in the lowest Sao_2 nadir during the TST (normal 94% +/− 2%, acyanotic 90% +/− 3%, and cyanotic 74% +/− 4% [$P<.01$]) and in the frequency distributions of percentage of TST with Sao_2 less than 90% (normal 10% +/− 17%, acyanotic 36% +/− 34%, and cyanotic 97% +/− 4% [$P<.05$]). Compared with the control group, the acyanotic group had a higher respiratory rate, lower tidal volume, and lower total respiratory compliance. Oxygen desaturation occurs during sleep in infants with CHD and seems related to the initial degree of hypoxemia and the presence of abnormal pulmonary function.

Patent foramen ovale (PFO) was detected in 27% to 69% of patients with documented OSA, suggesting a relationship between PFO and OSA, although with unclear relational pathophysiology. OSA has been postulated to induce right-to-left shunting through PFO via large swings in pleural pressure and pulmonary hypertension.[66]

The number of adults with CHD has increased due to advances in diagnosis and management, and SDB has been often observed in these patients. Although the report of SDB related morbidity is low in adults with CHD, in a review of perceived quality of life, those with CHD, especially single-ventricle physiology and cyanotic HD, reported poorer quality of work and sleep.[67]

In retrospective reviews of small cohort of adults with residual pulmonary incompetence after tetralogy of Fallot, Eisenmenger syndrome, and transposition of great arteries, varying degrees of sleep-related hypoxemia, significant desaturations, and SDB have been reported.[68–70] These lesions are also prone to right-sided chamber dilatation and dysfunction with risk of arrhythmia.[71] SDB is an important risk factor in the development of both pulmonary hypertension and atrial arrhythmia[72] and the dual risk may be detrimental. SDB may potentially complicate long-standing pulmonary incompetence due the effects of venous congestion on upper airway structures predisposing to OSA.[73] Because LV dysfunction is increasingly recognized in patients with a history of tetralogy of Fallot, CSA has also been noted.

The most common type of pulmonary hypertension diagnosed in childhood is pulmonary arterial hypertension (PAH) associated with CHD with a 5-year survival of 71%. The European Pediatric Pulmonary Vascular Disease Network recommends that patients with a suspicion or a predisposition for a breathing disorder (eg, patients with Down syndrome) and those with an inadequate response to PAH–targeted pharmacotherapy should undergo a formal sleep study, for diagnostic and direct therapeutic purposes.[74]

The effect of obesity in children with congenital heart disease

Approximately 17% of children ages 2 years to 19 years in the United States are obese, with an additional 15% who are considered overweight.[75] There is a strong correlation between obesity and the development of atherosclerotic disease even in childhood. Approximately 26% of children with congenital and acquired heart disease ages 6 years to 19 years had a BMI greater than 85% per Centers for Disease Control and Prevention criteria in a cohort from Philadelphia and Boston.[76] Systolic BP and BP percentiles were higher in obese and overweight patients with heart disease compared with those of normal weight.

Recent data from New York show that obesity and overweight affects approximately 30% of the pediatric CHD population,[77] and children of Hispanic ethnicity and male children were at the highest risk for development of obesity. The prevalence of obesity seems to increase in adulthood and approximately 54% of adults with CHD have a BMI greater than 25 kg/m^2.[78] This high prevalence of obesity may be related to traditional risk factors, such as genetic predisposition, sedentary lifestyle, poor dietary habits, and unique risk factors, such as higher caloric needs in early infancy and exercise restriction in childhood. Failure to thrive is a common symptom of heart failure in children with unrepaired heart defects and, therefore, maximizing caloric intake and encouraging weight gain are important in the overall health care in these at-risk children. Even though caloric requirements and metabolism normalize after cardiac repair, parents and health care providers often continue to emphasize increased caloric intake and weight gain and restriction from physical activity as a safety measure in the CHD population, both of which can ultimately lead to excessive weight gain and obesity. Formal activity restriction in children with CHD has been associated with higher BMI.[79]

Elevated nocturnal BP (an indicator of true systemic hypertension) and lower brachial artery reactivity (an indicator of endothelial dysfunction) have been observed in obese CHD children compared with normal-weight peers.[80] Obesity in the setting of CHD may have other important short-term and long-term implications as well. In a group of children with single ventricle physiology or those with CHD and CM who were listed for heart transplantation, pretransplant obesity is a significant risk factor for mortality. Patients with CHD often have underlying anatomic or functional abnormalities that cannot be altered by treatment and, therefore, obesity may be the only modifiable risk factor in this population.

Cardiomyopathy in Children

CM is rare in children, but it is a serious and life-threatening condition, with an annual incidence of 1.1/100,000 to 1.2/100,000.[81,82] Two-thirds of all pediatric CM cases are idiopathic, and the rest are either familial or secondary to neuromuscular disorders, myocarditis, malformation syndromes, and inborn errors of metabolism. The prognosis for children with CM is guarded, with high rates of morbidity and mortality.

In a prospective cross-sectional study, 21 patients with median age 10.7 years with CM (hypertrophic, dilated, and other), snoring was reported in 52% and SDB was observed in 48% patients. Significant CSA was noted in 24% of the cohort and in 50% of the SDB population. The LV end-diastolic volume index was greater in children with CSA than in children without SDB (P = .03). There were significant correlations between the central AHI and both LV end-diastolic and end-systolic volume indices.[83]

The hypothesized pathophysiology is that during sleep the rostral fluid shift from the limbs to the lungs and into the neck soft tissue causes excess fluid in the pulmonary interstitium, which stimulates the pulmonary irritant receptors, with resultant hyperventilation. Hyperventilation causes a lowering of CO_2 level below the apneic threshold, resulting in central apnea. OSA results from the excess accumulation of fluid around the neck and consequent upper-airway narrowing.

Duchenne muscular dystrophy

In patients with Duchenne muscular dystrophy (DMD), there is a bimodal distribution of SDB, with OSA affecting approximately 30% of the patients in the first decade of life and hypoventilation observed in the second decade.[84] Nocturnal hypoxemia is the first sign of respiratory failure due to sleep-related hypoventilation in REM sleep secondary to respiratory muscle weakness. The predominant cardiac manifestations are LV wall motion abnormalities, dilated CM, and pulmonary hypertension in those with nocturnal hypoxemia.[85]

Dilated and hypertrophic CM, arrhythmias, and conduction abnormalities, such as prolonged QT interval, have been reported in patients with dystrophinopathies.[86] In DMD patients, cardiac involvement develops insidiously during the first decade of life, often when skeletal muscle weakness is already significant. Sinus tachycardia is present in most patients after 5 years of age and persists throughout life. During the second decade of life, CM (hypertrophic and dilated) develops. The incidence of CM, especially dilated CM, is approximately 30% at 14 years of age and 50% at 18 years of age and is almost universal after 18 years of age.[87] Despite this high incidence, most patients with DMD remain asymptomatic probably because of a reduced cardiac workload in the wheelchair-bound state. Only 10% to 20% of DMD patients eventually die from cardiac disease. Patients with Becker muscular dystrophy (BMD), however, have worse prognosis, with congestive heart failure the most common cause of death. The postulated theory is that the slow progression of muscle weakness in BMD patients permits a prolonged workload on an impaired myocardium, which eventually results in dilated CM.[88]

The recommendations, therefore, are that DMD patients should undergo cardiac investigation at the time of diagnosis, before any surgery, every 2 years up to 10 years of age and annually thereafter.[88] Angiotensin-converting enzyme inhibitors and β-blockers may also slow the progression of the disease in DMD and systemic corticosteroids may also be protective. Cardiac transplantation is not an option in patients with DMD but may be an acceptable treatment in those with BMD.

OSA should be specifically treated in patients with DMD and bilevel positive airway pressure is recommended to correct nocturnal and daytime hypoventilation. In DMD patients, apart from medications for heart failure, the best treatment of Cheyne-Stokes respiration with central apnea due to congestive heart failure is uncertain and, therefore, supplemental oxygen, continuous positive airway pressure (CPAP) and bilevel positive airway pressure therapy may be considered.

Female DMD and BMD carriers have high incidence of cardiac involvement that progresses with age and manifests primarily as CM and, therefore, cardiac evaluation of DMD carriers is recommended every 5 years.[86]

Cardiac remodeling in obstructive sleep apnea in children

CM in children with SDB is most commonly described as LV diastolic dysfunction and hypertrophic CM.[89,90] Classically, children with OSA have been described as having RV dysfunction and pulmonary hypertension; however, lately several studies have shown LV involvement,[31,91] Increase in LV mass and relative wall thickness are found even in normotensive children with OSA.[91]

In children with OSA and adenotonsillar hypertrophy, cardiac abnormalities include LV end-diastolic dimension and increased thickness of interventricular septum. These changes have been showed to improve after adenotonsillectomy.[92,93] Nocturnal hypoxemia and inflammation have been reported to contribute to pathogenesis of cardiac remodeling and heart failure in children with OSA.[94–96] There is a need for larger and prospective studies to evaluate the timeline of development of cardiac abnormalities in patients with OSA.

Pediatric Heart Transplant

CHD and CM remain the most common indications for heart transplant in the infant age group (53%).[97] Chronic respiratory complications can occur after pediatric heart transplant, including OSA.[98,99]

In a retrospective review from the United Kingdom, lymphoid and gingival hyperplasia was noted in 8% of the heart transplant patients, and adenotonsillectomy and CPAP therapy were indicated for treatment of SDB.[98,100] Heart transplant recipients may be at an increased risk of the development of fatal ventricular arrhythmias if an allograft's response to hypoxia is suboptimal because of the delay in parasympathetic reinnervation of the allograft.[101]

Complete resolution of Cheyne-Stokes respirations with severe heart failure related to dilated CM after heart transplant has been reported in a 13-year-old patient.[102] A 10-year follow-up review of 42 infants who underwent heart transplantation revealed minimal incidence of SDB and an overall satisfactory quality of life, including sleep.[103]

New-onset restless legs syndrome after heart surgery in a child has been reported. It is postulated that the interaction between dysfunctional iron stores and intraoperative blood loss may have reduced the amount of brain iron triggering restless legs syndrome, along with immobilization and sleep deprivation after surgery.[104]

SLEEP AND CARDIOVASCULAR MORBIDITY IN SPECIFIC GENETIC SYNDROMES AND SYSTEMIC DISEASE IN CHILDREN
Down Syndrome

Down syndrome, or trisomy 21, is the most common known chromosomal disorder, with an incidence of 1 per 660 live births. OSA has a higher prevalence in children with Down syndrome (30% to 55%)[105] compared with healthy children (2%).[106] Patients with Down syndrome have

many predisposing risk factors for OSA, including midface and mandibular hypoplasia, glossoptosis, tonsillar and adenoidal hypertrophy, increased secretions, reduced tracheal diameter, and lower respiratory tract anomalies along with generalized hypotonia.

Approximately 40% of children who have Down syndrome have congenital cardiac lesions, including endocardial cushion defect, ventricular septal defect, and patent ductus arteriosus. OSA and nocturnal hypoxemia may contribute to pulmonary hypertension and cor pulmonale.[107]

OSA is an important cause of increased mortality in adults with Down syndrome[108] and the median age of death is 40 years. This is probably related to consequences of OSA, such as systemic arterial hypertension, pulmonary hypertension, right heart insufficiency, arrhythmias, and stroke,[109–111] and the risk increases in those with complications and sequelae from CHD. Pulmonary hypertension in children with Down syndrome may be reversed by relieving UAO.[48] New screening strategies for expected morbidities and treating them has improved the morbidity in patients with Down syndrome; however, the mortality rate is still high.

Achondroplasia

A majority of the skeletal dysplasias have anomalies affecting the chest wall and upper airway, placing these patients at higher risk for SDB and consequent CV complications.

The prevalence of achondroplasia is 1:1000 to 1:30,000 and is caused by mutations in FGFR-3 gene.[112] Clinical features include shortening of proximal limbs, short flared ribs, megalocephaly with short cranial base, small foramen magnum, and midface hypoplasia, and these predispose the patients to hypoxemia, hypoventilation, OSA, and central apnea[113–115] secondary to brainstem involvement. A recent study shwoed an AHI greater than 10 in 43% of study population.[115] Hypoxemia and OSA (16% of children with achondroplasia)[54] lead to pulmonary hypertension and RV hypertrophy or strain.[116]

Marfan Syndrome

Marfan syndrome occurs in 0.01% of general population and is caused by a defect in fibrillin-1.[117] The major cause of mortality is the aortic rupture secondary to aneurysm of thoracic aorta. OSA is found in 30% of patients and is a risk factor for aortic dilation; serial echocardiography is recommended to reduce mortality.[118,119] Retrognathia, increased neck circumference, and other facial anomalies can predispose these patients to developing OSA, thereby CV morbidities like pulmonary hypertension, diastolic dysfunction, heart failure, and systemic hypertension.[120]

Mucopolysaccharidosis

Mucopolysaccharidosis is a group of genetic disorders caused by defects in enzymes required for breakdown of glycosaminoglycans. The major manifestations are musculoskeletal and CV complications as seen in Hunter syndrome and Hurler syndrome. Patient with these syndromes have coarse facial features, macrocephaly, macroglossia, and cervical spine instability. Accumulation of mucopolysaccharides cause upper airway abnormalities, including thickening of the epiglottis and hypertrophy of adenoids and tonsils leading to OSA. The prevalence of OSA is 89% in mucopolysaccharidosis.[121–123] The CV morbidity seen is pulmonary hypertension, congestive heart failure, and cardiomyopathies secondary to mucopolysaccharide deposition in the cardiac muscle.[124,125] Recognizing and treating OSA will decrease the CV morbidity and mortality.[120]

Glycogen Storage Disorder

Glycogen storage disorders are genetic disorders with defective enzymes affecting the breakdown and synthesis of glycogen.[126] There are 11 subtypes; subtype 2 is Pompe disease. It is fatal in infants and presents with respiratory muscle weakness with hypoventilation.[127,128]

Pierre Robin Sequence

Pierre Robin sequence is a disorder that may occur singly or in association with Stickler syndrome, or 22q deletion. It consists of micrognathia, posterior displacement of the tongue and soft palate, and mandibular hypoplasia. Cardinal features include significant airway obstruction in the first few weeks of life warranting airway management. Severe airway obstruction can cause RV enlargement and dysfunction.[129]

CV abnormalities include CHD (40% of individuals), in particular conotruncal malformations (interrupted aortic arch [50%], persistent truncus arteriosus [34%], tetralogy of Fallot, and ventricular septal defect). Management strategies include tongue tip adhesion mandibular distraction, nasopharyngeal intubation, noninvasive positive pressure ventilation, or tracheostomy in severe cases.[130]

Apert Syndrome, Crouzon Syndrome, and Pfeiffer Syndrome

Apert syndrome, Crouzon syndrome, and Pfeiffer syndrome are genetic disorders involving mutation of FGFR-2 gene and are autosomal dominant inherited. Common features include craniosynostosis, maxillary hypoplasia, cleft palate, and tracheomalacia, which predispose OSA.[131,132] Unlike Pierre Robin sequence, the obstruction increases with growth and, therefore, serial monitoring and treatment of SDB are vital in this population.[133]

Sickle Cell Disease

Sickle cell disease (SCD) is a genetic disorder with autosomal recessive inheritance. The prevalence of SCD in African Americans is in 0.2%. Adults and children with SCD have shown to have nocturnal hypoxemia, systemic and pulmonary hypertension, and LV diastolic dysfunction.[134–137]

Recent studies have shown that children with SCD have unique restrictive CM superimposed on hyperdynamic physiology. This was characterized by diastolic dysfunction, left atrial dilation and normal systolic function and resulted in mild secondary pulmonary venous hypertension and elevated tricuspid regurgitation velocity, which may explain increased mortality and sudden death in patients with SCD.[138]

The prevalence of the OSA in patients with SCD is approximately 10%, which is higher than the general pediatric population (2%–5%).[139,140] Children with SCD may be at increased risk for the development of adenotonsillar hypertrophy as a compensatory response to functional asplenia or as a result of recurrent upper respiratory infections because of lack of opsonization of bacterial pathogens.[141] Decreased upper airway neuromuscular reflexes secondary to cerebral vasculopathy in SCD contribute to the increased upper airway collapsibility in children with SCD and OSA.[142]

Changes in LV afterload, intermittent hypoxemia, and recurrent arousals during sleep due to OSA lead to the development of LV hypertrophy, systemic hypertension, and cardiac remodeling, causing LV diastolic dysfunction in children and adults. Diastolic dysfunction precedes LV systolic impairment and, therefore, early recognition and appropriate therapy for LV diastolic dysfunction are recommended to reduce morbidity and mortality.[139]

SUMMARY

SDB is common in children secondary to multiple structural and physiologic causes. SDB often results in CV complications, especially when associated with other comorbidities. The bidirectional effect of CV pathologies causing SDB and SDB resulting in CV complications in children is discussed. Further review of available data and future prospective studies will help understand the prevalence of SDB and CV complications in children and help generate specific guidelines toward early diagnosis and management to improve quality of life and reduce morbidity and mortality.

REFERENCES

1. Chatow U, Davidson S, Reichman BL, et al. Development and maturation of the autonomic nervous system in premature and full-term infants using spectral analysis of heart rate fluctuations. Pediatr Res 1995;37(3):294–302.

2. Villa MP, Calcagnini G, Pagani J, et al. Effects of sleep stage and age on short-term heart rate variability during sleep in healthy infants and children. Chest 2000;117(2):460–6.

3. Mancia G, Baccelli G, Adams DB, et al. Vasomotor regulation during sleep in the cat. Am J Physiol 1971;220(4):1086–93.

4. Gassel MM, Ghelarducci B, Marchiafava PL, et al. Phasic changes in blood pressure and heart rate during the rapid eye movement episodes of desynchronized sleep in unrestrained cats. Arch Ital Biol 1964;102:530–44.

5. Guazzi M, Zanchetti A. Blood pressure and heart rate during natural sleep of cat and their regulation by carotid sinus and aortic reflexes. Arch Ital Biol 1965;103(4):789–817.

6. Kluge KA, Harper RM, Schechtman VL, et al. Spectral analysis assessment of respiratory sinus arrhythmia in normal infants and infants who subsequently died of sudden infant death syndrome. Pediatr Res 1988;24(6):677–82.

7. Liao D, Li X, Vgontzas AN, et al. Sleep-disordered breathing in children is associated with impairment of sleep stage-specific shift of cardiac autonomic modulation. J Sleep Res 2010;19(2):358–65.

8. Khositseth A, Chokechuleekorn J, Kuptanon T, et al. Rhythm disturbances in childhood obstructive sleep apnea during apnea-hypopnea episodes. Ann Pediatr Cardiol 2013;6(1):39–42.

9. El-Sheikh M, Erath SA, Bagley EJ. Parasympathetic nervous system activity and children's sleep. J Sleep Res 2013;22(3):282–8.

10. Iglayreger HB, Peterson MD, Liu D, et al. Sleep duration predicts cardiometabolic risk in obese adolescents. J Pediatr 2014;164(5):1085–90.e1.

11. Meininger JC, Gallagher MR, Eissa MA, et al. Sleep duration and its association with ambulatory blood pressure in a school-based, diverse sample of adolescents. Am J Hypertens 2014;27(7):948–55.

12. Spruyt K, Molfese DL, Gozal D. Sleep duration, sleep regularity, body weight, and metabolic homeostasis in school-aged children. Pediatrics 2011;127(2):e345–52.

13. Kaditis AG. Cardiovascular complications of childhood OSAS. In: Lenfant C, editor. Lung biology in health and disease, Volume 224. New York: Informa Healthcare; 2008.

14. Somers VK, Dyken ME, Mark AL, et al. Sympathetic-nerve activity during sleep in normal subjects. N Engl J Med 1993;328(5):303–7.

15. Somers VK, Dyken ME, Clary MP, et al. Sympathetic neural mechanisms in obstructive sleep apnea. J Clin Invest 1995;96(4):1897–904.

16. Coy TV, Dimsdale JE, Ancoli-Israel S, et al. Sleep apnoea and sympathetic nervous system activity: a review. J Sleep Res 1996;5(1):42–50.

17. O'Brien LM, Gozal D. Autonomic dysfunction in children with sleep-disordered breathing. Sleep 2005;28(6):747–52.

18. Baharav A, Kotagal S, Rubin BK, et al. Autonomic cardiovascular control in children with obstructive sleep apnea. Clin Auton Res 1999;9(6):345–51.

19. Minemura H, Akashiba T, Yamamoto H, et al. Acute effects of nasal continuous positive airway pressure on 24-hour blood pressure and catecholamines in patients with obstructive sleep apnea. Intern Med 1998;37(12):1009–13.

20. Marrone O, Riccobono L, Salvaggio A, et al. Catecholamines and blood pressure in obstructive sleep apnea syndrome. Chest 1993;103(3):722–7.

21. Marcus CL, Greene MG, Carroll JL. Blood pressure in children with obstructive sleep apnea. Am J Respir Crit Care Med 1998;157(4 Pt 1):1098–103.

22. Kohyama J, Ohinata JS, Hasegawa T. Blood pressure in sleep disordered breathing. Arch Dis Child 2003;88(2):139–42.

23. National High Blood Pressure Education Program Working Group on High Blood Pressure in Children and Adolescents. The fourth report on the diagnosis, evaluation, and treatment of high blood pressure in children and adolescents. Pediatrics 2004;114(2 Suppl 4th Report):555–76.

24. Leung LC, Ng DK, Lau MW, et al. Twenty-four-hour ambulatory BP in snoring children with obstructive sleep apnea syndrome. Chest 2006;130(4):1009–17.

25. Zintzaras E, Kaditis AG. Sleep-disordered breathing and blood pressure in children: a meta-analysis. Arch Pediatr Adolesc Med 2007;161(2):172–8.

26. Leuenberger U, Jacob E, Sweer L, et al. Surges of muscle sympathetic nerve activity during obstructive apnea are linked to hypoxemia. J Appl Physiol (1985) 1995;79(2):581–8.

27. Ringler J, Basner RC, Shannon R, et al. Hypoxemia alone does not explain blood pressure elevations after obstructive apneas. J Appl Physiol (1985) 1990;69(6):2143–8.

28. Amin RS, Kimball TR, Bean JA, et al. Left ventricular hypertrophy and abnormal ventricular geometry

in children and adolescents with obstructive sleep apnea. Am J Respir Crit Care Med 2002;165(10):1395–9.

29. Kaditis AG, Alexopoulos EI, Hatzi F, et al. Overnight change in brain natriuretic peptide levels in children with sleep-disordered breathing. Chest 2006;130(5):1377–84.

30. Sofer S, Weinhouse E, Tal A, et al. Cor pulmonale due to adenoidal or tonsillar hypertrophy or both in children. Noninvasive diagnosis and follow-up. Chest 1988;93(1):119–22.

31. Tal A, Leiberman A, Margulis G, et al. Ventricular dysfunction in children with obstructive sleep apnea: radionuclide assessment. Pediatr Pulmonol 1988;4(3):139–43.

32. Gileles-Hillel A, Alonso-Álvarez ML, Kheirandish-Gozal L, et al. Inflammatory markers and obstructive sleep apnea in obese children: the NANOS study. Mediators Inflamm 2014;2014:605280.

33. Kheirandish-Gozal L, Gileles-Hillel A, Alonso-Álvarez ML, et al. Effects of adenotonsillectomy on plasma inflammatory biomarkers in obese children with obstructive sleep apnea: a community-based study. Int J Obes (Lond) 2015;39(7):1094–100.

34. Maranduba CM, De Castro SB, de Souza GT, et al. Intestinal microbiota as modulators of the immune system and neuroimmune system: impact on the host health and homeostasis. J Immunol Res 2015;2015:931574.

35. Moreno-Indias I, Torres M, Montserrat JM, et al. Intermittent hypoxia alters gut microbiota diversity in a mouse model of sleep apnoea. Eur Respir J 2015;45(4):1055–65.

36. Kheirandish-Gozal L, Peris E, Wang Y, et al. Lipopolysaccharide-binding protein plasma levels in children: effects of obstructive sleep apnea and obesity. J Clin Endocrinol Metab 2014;99(2):656–63.

37. Hakim F, Kheirandish-Gozal L, Gozal D. Obesity and altered sleep: a pathway to metabolic derangements in children? Semin Pediatr Neurol 2015;22(2):77–85.

38. The AASM manual for the scoring of sleep and associated events, Version 2.3. Darien (IL): American Academy of Sleep Medicine; 2016.

39. Verhulst SL, Schrauwen N, Haentjens D, et al. Reference values for sleep-related respiratory variables in asymptomatic European children and adolescents. Pediatr Pulmonol 2007;42(2):159–67.

40. Uliel S, Tauman R, Greenfeld M, et al. Normal polysomnographic respiratory values in children and adolescents. Chest 2004;125(3):872–8.

41. Traeger N, Schultz B, Pollock AN, et al. Polysomnographic values in children 2-9 years old: additional data and review of the literature. Pediatr Pulmonol 2005;40(1):22–30.

42. Lanfranchi PA, Somers VK, Braghiroli A, et al. Central sleep apnea in left ventricular dysfunction: prevalence and implications for arrhythmic risk. Circulation 2003;107(5):727–32.

43. Javaheri S, Parker TJ, Liming JD, et al. Sleep apnea in 81 ambulatory male patients with stable heart failure. Types and their prevalences, consequences, and presentations. Circulation 1998;97(21):2154–9.

44. Eckert DJ, Jordan AS, Merchia P, et al. Central sleep apnea: pathophysiology and treatment. Chest 2007;131(2):595–607.

45. Khoo MC, Kronauer RE, Strohl KP, et al. Factors inducing periodic breathing in humans: a general model. J Appl Physiol Respir Environ Exerc Physiol 1982;53(3):644–59.

46. White DP. Pathogenesis of obstructive and central sleep apnea. Am J Respir Crit Care Med 2005;172(11):1363–70.

47. Wellman A, Malhotra A, Fogel RB, et al. Respiratory system loop gain in normal men and women measured with proportional-assist ventilation. J Appl Physiol (1985) 2003;94(1):205–12.

48. Dempsey JA. Crossing the apnoeic threshold: causes and consequences. Exp Physiol 2005;90(1):13–24.

49. Naughton M, Benard D, Tam A, et al. Role of hyperventilation in the pathogenesis of central sleep apneas in patients with congestive heart failure. Am Rev Respir Dis 1993;148(2):330–8.

50. Trinder J, Benard D, Tam A, et al. Pathophysiological interactions of ventilation, arousals, and blood pressure oscillations during cheyne-stokes respiration in patients with heart failure. Am J Respir Crit Care Med 2000;162(3 Pt 1):808–13.

51. Solin P, Roebuck T, Johns DP, et al. Peripheral and central ventilatory responses in central sleep apnea with and without congestive heart failure. Am J Respir Crit Care Med 2000;162(6):2194–200.

52. Kelly DH, Riordan L, Smith MJ. Apnea and periodic breathing in healthy full-term infants, 12-18 months of age. Pediatr Pulmonol 1992;13(3):169–71.

53. MacLean JE, Fitzgerald DA, Waters KA. Developmental changes in sleep and breathing across infancy and childhood. Paediatr Respir Rev 2015;16(4):276–84.

54. Zolty P, Sanders MH, Pollack IF. Chiari malformation and sleep-disordered breathing: a review of diagnostic and management issues. Sleep 2000;23(5):637–43.

55. Wolfe L, Lakadamyali H, Mutlu GM. Joubert syndrome associated with severe central sleep apnea. J Clin Sleep Med 2010;6(4):384–8.

56. Urquhart DS, Gulliver T, Williams G, et al. Central sleep-disordered breathing and the effects of oxygen therapy in infants with Prader-Willi syndrome. Arch Dis Child 2013;98(8):592–5.

57. Eichenwald EC, Committee on Fetus and Newborn, American Academy of Pediatrics. Apnea of prematurity. Pediatrics 2016;137(5).

58. Bagnall RD, Weintraub RG, Ingles J, et al. A prospective study of sudden cardiac death among children and young adults. N Engl J Med 2016;374(25):2441–52.

59. Myers MM, Gomez-Gribben E, Smith KS, et al. Developmental changes in infant heart rate responses to head-up tilting. Acta Paediatr 2006; 95(1):77–81.

60. Tuladhar R, Harding R, Adamson TM, et al. Heart rate responses to non-arousing trigeminal stimulation in infants: effects of sleep position, sleep state and postnatal age. Early Hum Dev 2005; 81(8):673–81.

61. Makielski JC. SIDS: genetic and environmental influences may cause arrhythmia in this silent killer. J Clin Invest 2006;116(2):297–9.

62. Weese-Mayer DE, Marazita ML, Rand CM, et al. Congenital central hypoventilation syndrome. In: Pagon RA, editor. GeneReviews(R). Seattle (WA): University of Washington; 1993.

63. Gronli JO, Santucci BA, Leurgans SE, et al. Congenital central hypoventilation syndrome: PHOX2B genotype determines risk for sudden death. Pediatr Pulmonol 2008;43(1):77–86.

64. Ykeda DS, Lorenzi-Filho G, Lopes AA, et al. Sleep in infants with congenital heart disease. Clinics (Sao Paulo) 2009;64(12):1205–10.

65. Hiatt PW, Mahony L, Tepper RS. Oxygen desaturation during sleep in infants and young children with congenital heart disease. J Pediatr 1992;121(2): 226–32.

66. Rigatelli G, Sharma S. Patent foramen ovale-obstructive sleep apnea relationships: pro and cons. Cardiovasc Revasc Med 2012;13(5):286–8.

67. Simko LC, McGinnis KA. What is the perceived quality of life of adults with congenital heart disease and does it differ by anomaly? J Cardiovasc Nurs 2005;20(3):206–14.

68. Hjortshoj CS, Jensen AS, Christensen JA, et al. Sleep-disordered breathing in eisenmenger syndrome. Int J Cardiol 2016;214:23–4.

69. Legault S, Lanfranchi P, Montplaisir J, et al. Nocturnal breathing in cyanotic congenital heart disease. Int J Cardiol 2008;128(2):197–200.

70. Cotts T, Smith KR, Lu J, et al. Risk for sleep-disordered breathing in adults after atrial switch repairs for d-looped transposition of the great arteries. Pediatr Cardiol 2014;35(5):888–92.

71. Gatzoulis MA, Balaji S, Webber SA, et al. Risk factors for arrhythmia and sudden cardiac death late after repair of tetralogy of Fallot: a multicentre study. Lancet 2000;356(9234):975–81.

72. Harrison DA, Siu SC, Hussain F, et al. Sustained atrial arrhythmias in adults late after repair of tetralogy of fallot. Am J Cardiol 2001;87(5):584–8.

73. Kasai T, Motwani SS, Yumino D, et al. Contrasting effects of lower body positive pressure on upper airways resistance and partial pressure of carbon dioxide in men with heart failure and obstructive or central sleep apnea. J Am Coll Cardiol 2013; 61(11):1157–66.

74. Lammers AE, Apitz C, Zartner P, et al. Diagnostics, monitoring and outpatient care in children with suspected pulmonary hypertension/paediatric pulmonary hypertensive vascular disease. Expert consensus statement on the diagnosis and treatment of paediatric pulmonary hypertension. The European Paediatric Pulmonary Vascular Disease Network, endorsed by ISHLT and DGPK. Heart 2016;102(Suppl 2):ii1–13.

75. Cohen MS. Clinical practice: the effect of obesity in children with congenital heart disease. Eur J Pediatr 2012;171(8):1145–50.

76. Pinto NM, Marino BS, Wernovsky G, et al. Obesity is a common comorbidity in children with congenital and acquired heart disease. Pediatrics 2007; 120(5):e1157–64.

77. Shustak RJ, McGuire SB, October TW, et al. Prevalence of obesity among patients with congenital and acquired heart disease. Pediatr Cardiol 2012; 33(1):8–14.

78. Pearson D, Rodriguez E, Fernandes S. Prevalence of obesity in adults with congenital heart disease. In: Program and abstracts of the fifth national conference of the adult congenital heart association. Philadelphia: PA; 2008.

79. Stefan MA, Hopman WM, Smythe JF. Effect of activity restriction owing to heart disease on obesity. Arch Pediatr Adolesc Med 2005;159(5):477–81.

80. Pasquali SK, Marino BS, Powell DJ, et al. Following the arterial switch operation, obese children have risk factors for early cardiovascular disease. Congenit Heart Dis 2010;5(1):16–24.

81. Lipshultz SE, Sleeper LA, Towbin JA, et al. The incidence of pediatric cardiomyopathy in two regions of the United States. N Engl J Med 2003;348(17): 1647–55.

82. Nugent AW, Daubeney PE, Chondros P, et al. The epidemiology of childhood cardiomyopathy in Australia. N Engl J Med 2003;348(17):1639–46.

83. Al-Saleh S, Kantor PF, Chadha NK, et al. Sleep-disordered breathing in children with cardiomyopathy. Ann Am Thorac Soc 2014;11(5):770–6.

84. Suresh S, Wales P, Dakin C, et al. Sleep-related breathing disorder in Duchenne muscular dystrophy: disease spectrum in the paediatric population. J Paediatr Child Health 2005;41(9–10): 500–3.

85. Melacini P, Vianello A, Villanova C, et al. Cardiac and respiratory involvement in advanced stage Duchenne muscular dystrophy. Neuromuscul Disord 1996;6(5):367–76.

86. Lemay J, Sériès F, Sénéchal M, et al. Unusual respiratory manifestations in two young adults with

Duchenne muscular dystrophy. Can Respir J 2012; 19(1):37–40.

87. Nigro G, Politano L, Nigro V, et al. Mutation of dystrophin gene and cardiomyopathy. Neuromuscul Disord 1994;4(4):371–9.

88. Bushby K, Muntoni F, Bourke JP. 107th ENMC international workshop: the management of cardiac involvement in muscular dystrophy and myotonic dystrophy. 7th-9th June 2002, Naarden, The Netherlands. Neuromuscul Disord 2003;13(2):166–72.

89. Sanchez-Armengol A, Rodríguez-Puras MJ, Fuentes-Pradera MA, et al. Echocardiographic parameters in adolescents with sleep-related breathing disorders. Pediatr Pulmonol 2003;36(1):27–33.

90. Bhattacharjee R, Kheirandish-Gozal L, Pillar G, et al. Cardiovascular complications of obstructive sleep apnea syndrome: evidence from children. Prog Cardiovasc Dis 2009;51(5):416–33.

91. Amin RS, Kimball TR, Kalra M, et al. Left ventricular function in children with sleep-disordered breathing. Am J Cardiol 2005;95(6):801–4.

92. Cincin A, Sakalli E, Bakirci EM, et al. Relationship between obstructive sleep apnea-specific symptoms and cardiac function before and after adenotonsillectomy in children with adenotonsillar hypertrophy. Int J Pediatr Otorhinolaryngol 2014;78(8):1281–7.

93. Weber SA, Pierri Carvalho R, Ridley G, et al. A systematic review and meta-analysis of cohort studies of echocardiographic findings in OSA children after adenotonsilectomy. Int J Pediatr Otorhinolaryngol 2014;78(10):1571–8.

94. Gozal D, Serpero LD, Kheirandish-Gozal L, et al. Sleep measures and morning plasma TNF-alpha levels in children with sleep-disordered breathing. Sleep 2010;33(3):319–25.

95. Tauman R, Ivanenko A, O'Brien LM, et al. Plasma C-reactive protein levels among children with sleep-disordered breathing. Pediatrics 2004; 113(6):e564–9.

96. Robinson GV, Pepperell JC, Segal HC, et al. Circulating cardiovascular risk factors in obstructive sleep apnoea: data from randomised controlled trials. Thorax 2004;59(9):777–82.

97. Dipchand AI, Rossano JW, Edwards LB, et al. The registry of the international society for heart and lung transplantation: eighteenth official pediatric heart transplantation Report–2015; focus theme: early graft failure. J Heart Lung Transplant 2015; 34(10):1233–43.

98. Thomas B, Flet JG, Shyam R, et al. Chronic respiratory complications in pediatric heart transplant recipients. J Heart Lung Transplant 2007;26(3):236–40.

99. Klink ME, Sethi GK, Copeland JG, et al. Obstructive sleep apnea in heart transplant patients. A report of five cases. Chest 1993;104(4):1090–2.

100. Homma S, Takahashi K, Nihei S, et al. The successful management of respiratory complications with long-term, low-dose macrolide administration in pediatric heart transplant recipients. Int Heart J 2014;55(6):560–3.

101. Madden BP, Shenoy V, Dalrymple-Hay M, et al. Absence of bradycardic response to apnea and hypoxia in heart transplant recipients with obstructive sleep apnea. J Heart Lung Transplant 1997; 16(4):394–7.

102. Al-Saleh S, Kantor PF, Narang I. Impact of heart transplantation on cheyne-stokes respiration in a child. Case Rep Pediatr 2016;2016:4698756.

103. Gandhi SK, Canter CE, Kulikowska A, et al. Infant heart transplantation ten years later–where are they now? Ann Thorac Surg 2007;83(1):169–71 [discussion: 172].

104. Cortese S, Konofal E, Lecendreux M, et al. Restless legs syndrome triggered by heart surgery. Pediatr Neurol 2006;35(3):223–6.

105. de Miguel-Diez J, Villa-Asensi JR, Alvarez-Sala JL. Prevalence of sleep-disordered breathing in children with Down syndrome: polygraphic findings in 108 children. Sleep 2003;26(8):1006–9.

106. Redline S, Tishler PV, Schluchter M, et al. Risk factors for sleep-disordered breathing in children. Associations with obesity, race, and respiratory problems. Am J Respir Crit Care Med 1999;159(5 Pt 1):1527–32.

107. Loughlin GM, Wynne JW, Victorica BE. Sleep apnea as a possible cause of pulmonary hypertension in Down syndrome. J Pediatr 1981;98(3): 435–7.

108. He J, Kryger MH, Zorick FJ, et al. Mortality and apnea index in obstructive sleep apnea. Experience in 385 male patients. Chest 1988;94(1):9–14.

109. Mohsenin V. Sleep-related breathing disorders and risk of stroke. Stroke 2001;32(6):1271–8.

110. Young T, Peppard PE, Gottlieb DJ. Epidemiology of obstructive sleep apnea: a population health perspective. Am J Respir Crit Care Med 2002; 165(9):1217–39.

111. Yang Q, Rasmussen SA, Friedman JM. Mortality associated with Down's syndrome in the USA from 1983 to 1997: a population-based study. Lancet 2002;359(9311):1019–25.

112. Richette P, Bardin T, Stheneur C. Achondroplasia: from genotype to phenotype. Joint Bone Spine 2008;75(2):125–30.

113. Mogayzel PJ Jr, Carroll JL, Loughlin GM, et al. Sleep-disordered breathing in children with achondroplasia. J Pediatr 1998;132(4):667–71.

114. Julliand S, Boulé M, Baujat G, et al. Lung function, diagnosis, and treatment of sleep-disordered breathing in children with achondroplasia. Am J Med Genet A 2012;158A(8):1987–93.

115. Afsharpaiman S, Saburi A, Waters KA. Respiratory difficulties and breathing disorders in achondroplasia. Paediatr Respir Rev 2013;14(4):250–5.

116. Wynn J, King TM, Gambello MJ, et al. Mortality in achondroplasia study: a 42-year follow-up. Am J Med Genet A 2007;143A(21):2502–11.

117. Loeys B, De Backer J, Van Acker P, et al. Comprehensive molecular screening of the FBN1 gene favors locus homogeneity of classical Marfan syndrome. Hum Mutat 2004;24(2):140–6.

118. Kohler M, Blair E, Risby P, et al. The prevalence of obstructive sleep apnoea and its association with aortic dilatation in Marfan's syndrome. Thorax 2009;64(2):162–6.

119. Kohler M, Pitcher A, Blair E, et al. The impact of obstructive sleep apnea on aortic disease in Marfan's syndrome. Respiration 2013;86(1):39–44.

120. Shahar E, Whitney CW, Redline S, et al. Sleep-disordered breathing and cardiovascular disease: cross-sectional results of the Sleep Heart Health Study. Am J Respir Crit Care Med 2001;163(1):19–25.

121. Semenza GL, Pyeritz RE. Respiratory complications of mucopolysaccharide storage disorders. Medicine (Baltimore) 1988;67(4):209–19.

122. Shapiro J, Strome M, Crocker AC. Airway obstruction and sleep apnea in Hurler and Hunter syndromes. Ann Otol Rhinol Laryngol 1985;94(5 Pt 1):458–61.

123. Muenzer J. The mucopolysaccharidoses: a heterogeneous group of disorders with variable pediatric presentations. J Pediatr 2004;144(5 Suppl):S27–34.

124. Belani KG, Krivit W, Carpenter BL, et al. Children with mucopolysaccharidosis: perioperative care, morbidity, mortality, and new findings. J Pediatr Surg 1993;28(3):403–8 [discussion: 408–10].

125. Martins AM, Dualibi AP, Norato D, et al. Guidelines for the management of mucopolysaccharidosis type I. J Pediatr 2009;155(4 Suppl):S32–46.

126. Hers HG. alpha-Glucosidase deficiency in generalized glycogenstorage disease (Pompe's disease). Biochem J 1963;86:11–6.

127. Kansagra S, Austin S, DeArmey S, et al. Longitudinal polysomnographic findings in infantile Pompe disease. Am J Med Genet A 2015;167A(4):858–61.

128. Kishnani PS, Hwu WL, Mandel H, et al. A retrospective, multinational, multicenter study on the natural history of infantile-onset Pompe disease. J Pediatr 2006;148(5):671–6.

129. Spier S, Rivlin J, Rowe RD, et al. Sleep in pierre robin syndrome. Chest 1986;90(5):711–5.

130. Cote A, Fanous A, Almajed A, et al. Pierre Robin sequence: review of diagnostic and treatment challenges. Int J Pediatr Otorhinolaryngol 2015;79(4):451–64.

131. Mixter RC, David DJ, Perloff WH, et al. Obstructive sleep apnea in Apert's and Pfeiffer's syndromes: more than a craniofacial abnormality. Plast Reconstr Surg 1990;86(3):457–63.

132. Cohen MM Jr, Kreiborg S. Upper and lower airway compromise in the Apert syndrome. Am J Med Genet 1992;44(1):90–3.

133. Driessen C, Joosten KF, Bannink N, et al. How does obstructive sleep apnoea evolve in syndromic craniosynostosis? A prospective cohort study. Arch Dis Child 2013;98(7):538–43.

134. Sachdev V, Kato GJ, Gibbs JS, et al. Echocardiographic markers of elevated pulmonary pressure and left ventricular diastolic dysfunction are associated with exercise intolerance in adults and adolescents with homozygous sickle cell anemia in the United States and United Kingdom. Circulation 2011;124(13):1452–60.

135. Gladwin MT, Sachdev V. Cardiovascular abnormalities in sickle cell disease. J Am Coll Cardiol 2012;59(13):1123–33.

136. Sachdev V, Kato GJ, Gibbs JS, et al. Diastolic dysfunction is an independent risk factor for death in patients with sickle cell disease. J Am Coll Cardiol 2007;49(4):472–9.

137. Gladwin MT, Sachdev V, Jison ML, et al. Pulmonary hypertension as a risk factor for death in patients with sickle cell disease. N Engl J Med 2004;350(9):886–95.

138. Niss O, Quinn CT, Lane A, et al. Cardiomyopathy with restrictive physiology in sickle cell disease. JACC Cardiovasc Imaging 2016;9(3):243–52.

139. Rosen CL, Debaun MR, Strunk RC, et al. Obstructive sleep apnea and sickle cell anemia. Pediatrics 2014;134(2):273–81.

140. Sharma S, Efird JT, Knupp C, et al. Sleep disorders in adult sickle cell patients. J Clin Sleep Med 2015;11(3):219–23.

141. Strauss T, Sin S, Marcus CL, et al. Upper airway lymphoid tissue size in children with sickle cell disease. Chest 2012;142(1):94–100.

142. Huang J, Pinto SJ, Allen JL, et al. Upper airway genioglossal activity in children with sickle cell disease. Sleep 2011;34(6):773–8.

Rehabilitation of Cardiovascular Disorders and Sleep Apnea

Behrouz Jafari, MD[a,b],*

KEYWORDS

- Obstructive sleep apnea • Sleep disordered breathing • Cardiac rehabilitation
- Stroke rehabilitation • Cardiovascular disease • Stroke

KEY POINTS

- Obstructive sleep apnea (OSA) is a common disorder in patients entering cardiac rehabilitation units.
- Sleep disordered breathing is underdiagnosed in the poststroke period.
- Early screening and treatment of OSA are important in the management of the poststroke period or after cardiac events.
- Failure to treat OSA in cardiac patients and patients with stroke can have negative impacts on outcomes during rehabilitation.

INTRODUCTION

Obstructive sleep apnea (OSA) syndrome is a disorder affecting 2% to 4% of the general population in the United States.[1–3] It is characterized by recurrent episodes of upper airway collapse during sleep. This condition presents in more than half of patients with acute coronary heart disease who are eligible for enrollment in cardiac rehabilitation programs.[4] Because of the hemodynamic fluctuations associated with OSA, those patients with concurrent OSA who enter cardiac rehabilitation programs may be placed at greater risk for arrhythmias and exercise-related complications.[5] This risk can lead to an increase in major adverse cardiac events such as revascularization, heart failure (HF), hospital readmission, functional limitation, and reduced quality of life in cardiac patients.

In contrast, stroke, with an incidence of 2 to 18 per 1000 per year, is the second leading cause of death worldwide and more than 50% of survivors have mental and physical impairment.[6,7] Although sleep disordered breathing (SDB) has been recognized in patients with stroke since the early nineteenth century,[8] over the last 2 decades it has been emerging as an important cardiovascular risk factor.

In the poststroke period, patients with OSA have greater disability and higher mortality than patients without OSA.[9,10] However, OSA is under-recognized during the poststroke period because of a lack of symptoms or lack of gross obesity, despite evidence that managing this risk factor may benefit those patients.[11] There is growing evidence that treatment of coexisting OSA with continuous positive airway pressure (CPAP) or mandibular advancement devices can successfully treat OSA, resulting in improved rehabilitation outcomes and improved health-related quality of life.[12–15]

Disclosure: The author has nothing to disclose.
[a] Section of Pulmonary, Critical Care and Sleep Medicine, School of Medicine, University of California-Irvine, 333 City Boulevard West, Suite 400, Irvine, CA, USA; [b] Sleep Program, VA Long Beach Healthcare System, 5901 East 7th Street, Long Beach, CA 90822, USA
* Sleep Program, VA Long Beach Healthcare System, 5901 East 7th Street, Long Beach, CA.
E-mail address: jafarib@uci.edu

sleep.theclinics.com

PREVALENCE OF OBSTRUCTIVE SLEEP APNEA IN PATIENTS ENTERING CARDIAC REHABILITATION PROGRAMS

It is well known that patients with different types of cardiovascular diseases have higher prevalence of SDB.[16–19] Several studies have shown that OSA is an independent risk factor for development of hypertension and has a dose-response relationship between severity of OSA and incidence of hypertension.[18,20,21] SDB is also estimated to have a prevalence of 30% to 69% in patients with coronary artery disease (CAD)[22–24] and 50% to 70% in patients with systolic HF.[25,26] However, fewer data are available in HF with preserved ejection fraction (EF) than in those with reduced EF. The largest study on this group was done on 244 consecutive patients: 97 patients (39.8%) presented with OSA and 72 patients (29.5%) with central sleep apnea (CSA).[27]

In the postdischarge period after coronary revascularization procedures, 52% to 64%[28,29] of patients had moderate to severe OSA. A recent study suggested that, overall, 53% of patients entering cardiac rehabilitation programs are at high risk, or are previously diagnosed with OSA.[4] However, the experts believe that the prevalence of OSA is substantially higher and is largely under-recognized in patients entering cardiac rehabilitation programs.[30]

PREVALENCE OF OBSTRUCTIVE SLEEP APNEA IN THE POSTSTROKE PERIOD

In the past decade, longitudinal studies have shown that people with SDB have a greater risk for stroke.[31–35] The reported prevalence in the literature is very high, ranging from 40% to 90%,[9,10,34,36–40] likely reflecting different study designs and definitions of SDB.

Yaggi and colleagues[41] followed 1022 patients over 6 years and found that OSA is associated with an increased risk for stroke, transient ischemic attack, and death. This finding was true even after adjusting for age, gender, body mass index (BMI), arterial hypertension, diabetes, atrial fibrillation, hyperlipidemia, and smoking habits. Patients with severe SDB had a higher chance of having stroke (hazard ratio [HR], 3.3; confidence interval [CI], 1.7–6.3). These results were confirmed by other investigators as well.[35,42–44]

It has been shown that many patients experience a recurrent stroke within 5 years of their first attack[45] and those with recurrent stroke have a higher chance of having SDB compared with first-time stroke victims.[46] Note that presence of an apnea-hypopnea index (AHI) greater than 10

per hour is an independent risk factor for stroke recurrence.[46]

The prevalence of sleep apnea is highest early following stroke and may decrease during recovery,[34,47] reflecting a decrease in sleep apnea in most patients, although it can also be caused by a higher mortality in those with more severe form of disease. Although SDB tends to improve spontaneously several weeks after stroke, approximately 50% of patients still have OSA 3 months after the acute event.[31,32,34] Szücs and colleagues[48] reported that the frequency and severity of sleep apnea were unchanged 3 months later in most patients with ischemic stroke, whereas it was greatly improved in patients with hemorrhagic stroke. Moreover, hemorrhagic strokes lead more often to central apneas.[49]

Both OSA and, less frequently, CSA have been identified as risk factors for stroke.[10] However, only OSA is recognized as a mortality risk for ischemic stroke.[9,48,49] Periodic breathing (PB) may also develop in patients with stroke in the absence of cardiopulmonary disease, disturbed consciousness, or HF.[50] During the acute phase of stroke, obstructive apnea is the most predominant type. Central apneas are associated with altered mental status, brain edema, and ischemia of brainstem and their incidence diminishes during recovery after stroke.[51] Rowat and colleagues[52] investigated the impact of PB in the awake state on mortality in the immediate phase after stroke. They investigated 138 patients with stroke at a median of 4 hours after stroke and found that those with PB were more likely to have severe stroke and more likely to be dead or dependent at 3 months. In contrast, another study showed that CSA was not related to early death among the patients with stroke. Only patients with OSA (AHI >10) had an increased risk of early death.[9]

In a prospective study on 161 patients admitted to a stroke unit, no relationships were found between sleep-related respiratory events and the topographic location of the neurologic lesion or vascular involvement.[34]

WHY OBSTRUCTIVE SLEEP APNEA IS UNDER-RECOGNIZED IN STROKE AND CARDIAC REHABILITATION UNITS

OSA is rarely considered in rehabilitation units despite evidence that managing OSA, when present, may benefit patients with cardiovascular diseases. It has been shown that, despite higher prevalence of SDB among patients with stroke, none of them had been referred for diagnostic studies because SDB had not been suspected clinically because of less sleepiness and lower BMI.

The late diagnosis of sleep apnea can potentially have a negative impact on the outcomes and rehabilitation processes of these patients.[11] Two key clinical symptoms, excessive daytime sleepiness and obesity, do not seem to be prevalent in patients after stroke[10,13,53,54] or HF.[55] Bassetti and colleagues[53] showed that those with ischemic strokes were neither obese nor sleepy despite having severe OSA. They reported that 26 out of 152 patients with stroke had severe OSA with an AHI greater than or equal to 30, but their mean Epworth Sleepiness Scale(ESS) score was 6 and BMI of 27.9 kg/m^2 indicated that they were not obese and did not have excessive daytime sleepiness.[53] Similarly, Wessendorf and colleagues[56] showed that, in 105 patients with stroke and moderate to severe OSA (AHI $\geq$15), the mean ESS score was 7 and mean BMI was 28.7 kg/m^2. Kaneko and colleagues[10] made similar observations as well (mean ESS score of 5 and BMI of 28.8 kg/m^2).

The ESS relies on the self-perception of sleepiness. In patients without stroke and cardiovascular disease, the ESS correlates modestly, but significantly, with the AHI and with objective measures of sleepiness such as the Multiple Sleep Latency Test[57] and the Oxford Sleep Resistance Test.[55] There are several possibilities that might explain the lack of sleepiness in patients with stroke, including cognitive impairment, low physical activity, or drug-related factors.[54,58,59] In one study, patients with stroke were only mildly impaired and there was no significant relationship between Mini-Mental State Examination and ESS scores.[54] This finding indicates that cognitive impairment probably is not the reason for the lack of reported daytime sleepiness.

Another proposed potential explanation for the lower ESS scores in patients with stroke is low level of physical activity, so they may be less likely to feel sleepy.[54] The investigators suggest that most of their physical needs are met by hospital personnel, and as a result they are less physically active, which might affect subjective sleepiness.[54] Although it seems a plausible reason, there is no evidence to accept this as the cause of less daytime sleepiness.

Another possible reason is that drugs commonly used in patients with cardiac disease, such as β-receptor blockers, diuretics, statins, thrombocyte aggregation inhibitors, and antiarrhythmics, may cause a reduced perception of daytime sleepiness through a central nervous system–stimulating effect. However, none of them are known to have such effects, and none have been reported to reduce perception of sleepiness.[60] Therefore, it is unlikely that these drugs could explain lower levels of sleepiness in patients with stroke.

These findings in patients with stroke are similar to those previously described in cardiovascular patients, who also had less daytime sleepiness at any given OSA severity.[58,59] Arzt and colleagues[54] reported that patients with HF with any OSA severity had lower mean ESS (7), indicating less sleepiness despite sleeping less. This finding in patients with HF shows that the absence of subjective sleepiness is not a reliable means of ruling out OSA.[55]

Another finding was the lack of an association between BMI and the severity of OSA in patients with stroke, which contrasts with the well-established relationship between increasing BMI and increasing severity of OSA in patients without stroke.[61,62]

All of the studies discussed earlier showed that lower ESS scores and BMI in patients with stroke or HF and OSA cannot be explained by differences in the severity of OSA or other confounding factors and that those are not sensitive independent predictors of the presence of OSA.[63]

Therefore, regardless of the underlying mechanisms, lower ESS scores and BMI may make the diagnosis of OSA less likely in the rehabilitation period, and as a result may have a negative impact on clinical course and outcome.

OBSTRUCTIVE SLEEP APNEA AND REHABILITATION OUTCOME

Stroke and cardiac rehabilitation programs combine physical rehabilitation with education, self-management, and psychological support. The goal of postacute rehabilitation is to facilitate return home by assisting patients in achieving independence in personal care activities. In addition, it provides an opportunity to identify any comorbidity such as hypertension, and diabetes that may delay recovery. Therefore, early recognition and treatment of OSA during acute rehabilitation should be important parts of recovery. There is growing evidence that failure to treat OSA in cardiac patients can have a negative effect on postoperative recovery and increase mortality and morbidity, reduce quality of life, and lead to worse outcomes during and after the cardiac rehabilitation.[64,65] Hargenes and colleagues[66] studied patients entering an early outpatient cardiac rehabilitation program and found that cardiac patients with OSA had significantly lower cardiac output, stroke volume, and contractility index. They suggested that the decreased cardiac function in the OSA group, likely because of pressure and volume alteration associated with apneic events, may place these patients at a disadvantage in recovering from their cardiac events, and at increased risk for secondary complications.

In a recent study in which 67 consecutive patients referred for coronary artery bypass grafting (CABG) underwent clinical evaluation and were followed for a mean of 4.5 years after CABG, 56% of patients had moderate-severe OSA.[67] Those with sleep apnea had significantly higher major adverse cardiac or cerebrovascular events (35% vs 16%; $P = .02$) and new revascularization (19% vs 0%; $P = .01$). OSA was an independent factor associated with these events in the multivariate analysis.[67]

In a prospective observational study, patients with acute myocardial infarction (MI) and percutaneous coronary intervention underwent cardiovascular magnetic resonance to define salvaged myocardium and infarct size within 3 to 5 days and at 3 months after acute MI. Of the 56 patients included, 29 (52%) had SDB. Patients with SDB had significantly less salvaged myocardium, smaller reduction in infarct size within 3 months after acute MI, a larger final infarct size, and a lower final left ventricular EF.[28] In a multivariate analysis, including established risk factors for large MI, AHI was independently associated with less myocardial salvage and a larger infarct size 3 months after acute MI.[28]

In contrast, the presence of OSA in the setting of stroke is associated with unfavorable clinical course, including early neurologic worsening, delirium, depressed mood, impaired functional capacity and cognition, longer period of hospitalization and rehabilitation, and increased mortality.[1,7,9,10,36,37,68–72] In addition, severe OSA not only increases the risk of stroke recurrence but also increases the incidence of fatal and nonfatal cardiovascular events as well as sudden death during sleep.[44,73–75] The higher blood pressure and its swing during episodes of upper airways obstruction lead to worse outcome following stroke.[76] Sleep apnea probably promotes this functional impairment through intermittent nocturnal hypoxia, reduced cerebral perfusion, and fragmented sleep.[77]

Sleep quality can influence the rehabilitation process. The development of poor sleep with frequent arousals may be particularly important and persist long after stroke symptoms have resolved. In addition, poor sleep quality might have a negative impact on patients' motivation, level of energy, and participation in rehabilitation. Prior study suggests that SDB and poor sleep during rehabilitation were associated with less functional recovery between admission and discharge.[37,78] This association can persist up to 3 months after admission[78] and persisted when analyses were adjusted for other significant independent predictors of functional recovery, including total hours of therapy received, mental status, acute hospital transfer during the rehabilitation stay, and reason for admission to rehabilitation facility.[78] This finding is particularly important because, although many other predictors of rehabilitation outcomes are difficult or impossible to change, abnormal sleep pattern can be a modifiable predictor of rehabilitation outcomes. Interventions to improve abnormal sleep/wake patterns and early treatment of SDB during rehabilitation may result in better functional recovery among older people. Studies in other institutional settings (eg, nursing homes, acute care hospitals) suggest that sleep problems are associated with social isolation, poor health, and functional impairment in older people.[79–83] Those with excessive daytime sleepiness required more assistance with self-care activities, engaged in fewer social interactions,[82,83] and showed worse health-related quality of life.[84] In addition, they had slower recovery of functional abilities and longer stay in rehabilitation units.[10,85] These outcomes can lead to increased caregiving needs at home, nursing home placement, or death,[86] and may have detrimental effects on rehabilitation[64,87] and long-term outcome.[88]

Functional independence in personal care activities can be measured using the motor subscale of the Functional Independence Measure (mFIM),[89] which is widely used in rehabilitation settings to assess functional limitations and changes in functional status with rehabilitation therapy. Prior work suggests that a 1-point improvement in mFIM score is associated with 2.2 fewer minutes of help required from another person each day,[90] which translates into 15 minutes of caregiving per week for every 1-point change in mFIM. Every 10% reduction in daytime sleepiness is associated with 1-point additional improvement in mFIM during rehabilitation.[78] This degree of change in daytime sleepiness is achievable by using interventions to improve sleep patterns. It was also associated with increased participation in social and physical activities.[82] This relationship between more daytime sleepiness and less favorable immediate-term and long-term functional recovery suggests that sleep is an important modifiable predictor of rehabilitation outcomes for this vulnerable patient population.

Good and colleagues[37] found that patients with recent stroke and sleep apnea had poorer functional outcomes assessed with the Barthel Activities of Daily Living (ADL) index at discharge from rehabilitation as well as 3 and 12 months after stroke onset. Soon after admission to the stroke rehabilitation unit, these patients are more dependent in their ADLs and have longer latency in reaction and in response to verbal stimuli, impairing their ability to acquire new skills.[14] In addition, the presence of SDB was associated with a worse Barthel index at 6 months after stroke[91] and predicted a higher mortality during the following 10 years.[9,53,91] Note that high mortality was found only in patients with OSA but not CSA.[9]

Other symptoms in patients with stroke and cardiac disorders are impaired memory, lack of ability to concentrate, and tiredness, which are common in patients with OSA.[92,93] These patients are less adherent to rehabilitation programs because of decreased functional capacity[94] and depression.[64,87] Poor sleep and fatigue are associated with neuropsychiatric and cognitive disturbances, and result in worse outcomes in rehabilitation and quality of life.[95] Depression after stroke occurs in 30% to 60% of patients with stroke[96] and poor sleep strongly correlates with health complaints and depressive symptoms.[97] Previous studies have shown that depression and cognitive impairment commonly occur in patients with sleep apnea but without stroke, and improve after CPAP treatment.[98–100] This finding indicates that emotional instability in this population might be sleep related and therefore it is reasonable to consider and investigate the SDB, if other symptoms exist.

Poststroke fatigue is an independent predictor of dependency and death. In a cohort study of 8194 patients with stroke,[101] 39% of patients reported fatigue 2 years after their stroke. Patients with fatigue were more likely to be institutionalized and had increased mortality in the subsequent year.[101]

In some studies, delirium was reported in up to half of patients, especially in the first week after ischemic stroke.[102,103] This delirium can prolong hospital stay and increases risk of dementia and admission to an institution.[103,104] Well-known risk factors for delirium are hypoxemia[105] and OSA, which can be reversed by CPAP treatment.[106–108]

These studies show high prevalence of OSA at different time points from stroke onset or cardiac event and OSA exerts a negative effect on the functional recovery of these patients. Therefore, patients with cardiovascular diseases should be screened for OSA early in the course of their disease.

However, the question remains whether early intervention for treatment of OSA shortly after stroke or cardiac event alters the neurologic recovery and/or outcome.

EARLY TREATMENT OF OBSTRUCTIVE SLEEP APNEA IN STROKE REHABILITATION

The central nervous system is very sensitive to hypoperfusion in the poststroke period. Therefore, interventions designed to improve poststroke functioning are more effective the earlier they are delivered after symptom onset to reduce mortality and disability. Upper airway obstruction presents a potential therapeutic target to improve outcomes, because control of sleep apnea may prevent hypoxemia, large fluctuations in blood pressure, and cerebral hypoperfusion. To address this, previous studies have examined the potential beneficial effects of OSA treatment on neurologic and cognitive functions of patients during the stable phase of stroke in a rehabilitation setting. Bravata and colleagues[47] randomized 55 patients to an intervention group (stroke standard of care plus auto-CPAP) and control group (only stroke standard of care). Patients with stroke randomized to the intervention group received 2 nights of auto-CPAP, but only those with evidence of OSA received auto-CPAP for the remainder of the 30-day period. Change in stroke severity was assessed by comparing the National Institutes of Health (NIH) Stroke Scale (NIHSS) score at baseline versus at 30 days. Intervention patients had greater improvements in NIHSS score (−3.0) than control patients (−1.0; $P = .03$). Among patients with OSA, greater improvement was observed with increasing auto-CPAP use.

In another randomized study on 50 patients with stroke,[109] CPAP use within 24 hours of hospitalization resulted in a significant improvement in the NIHSS score. In both trials, greater improvement was noted with increasing CPAP use.

Both sleep apnea and blood pressure variability confer a poor prognosis after stroke and are potentially treatable.[76] Treatment of coexisting OSA decreases both nocturnal and diurnal blood pressure[56,110] and as a result reduces risk of stroke recurrence,[111] reduces mortality,[74] and improves quality of life.[56,69] Because SDB improves after the acute phase of stroke, auto-CPAP systems may be preferable.[47,112]

Among the most prominent potential benefits of CPAP therapy are motor and functional outcomes. However, randomized controlled trials were not strong enough to show this effect. Some studies found that CPAP improved 1 or more neurologic function outcomes, sleepiness, or mood,[13–15,47] whereas the others found no benefit of CPAP treatment in these areas.[113–115] However, the negative studies had small sample sizes and patients had low CPAP compliance, which may have affected the results.

One of the obstacles of OSA treatment in the stroke population has been poor compliance. There are several reasons for poor compliance, including spontaneous improvement of SDB, lack of excessive daytime sleepiness in some patients, and motor (facial and bulbar palsy) and cognitive (confusional states, dementia, aphasia) deficits. Compliance has been reported to be as low as 25% to 50% in the acute[39,53,113,116,117] or subacute[69,74,114] stroke phase, whereas other groups reported rates as high as 70% in the rehabilitation setting.[56] This finding indicates the importance of CPAP acclimation by skilled respiratory therapists.

In summary, previous research suggests that treatment of OSA with CPAP improves functional recovery during stroke rehabilitation, but that the effect of CPAP treatment on cognitive function in patients with stroke is still unclear.

EARLY TREATMENT OF OBSTRUCTIVE SLEEP APNEA IN CARDIOVASCULAR REHABILITATION

Before the availability of CPAP, the only known definitive therapy for OSA was tracheostomy. One of the earliest studies that showed the impact of treatment of OSA was a retrospective cohort in the 1970s.[118] There were 198 patients followed for 7 years. Seventy-one patients received tracheostomy and 127 received conservative treatment consisting of recommended weight loss. The tracheostomy group (as curative treatment) developed considerably fewer vascular complications.[118] Another observational cohort study examined the impact of CPAP on long-term cardiovascular outcomes in patients with sleep apnea and showed that CPAP therapy reduces fatal and nonfatal cardiovascular events and protected against death from cardiovascular disease.[44,119,120]

Short-term randomized trials have been studying systemic blood pressure as the outcome. Although the results have been different with respect to the magnitude of blood pressure reduction, it seems to be a clinically important blood pressure reduction. Those studies showed that patients who had more severe and symptomatic sleep apnea and hypertension experienced more benefit from the longer use of CPAP.[110,121,122] Patients less likely to experience benefit were those with asymptomatic mild OSA who had normal blood pressure at baseline.[123,124] In a double-blind, randomized trial comparing therapeutic airway pressurization with sham CPAP, therapeutic airway pressurization was associated with a reduction of 3 to 7 mm Hg in mean 24-hour systemic arterial blood pressure.[122] In extrapolating from pharmacologic antihypertensive trials, this blood pressure reduction, in itself, is expected to result in a 20% stroke risk reduction.[125]

To date, there are very few data available about the treatment of OSA in the context of cardiac rehabilitation and, overall, the data supporting the treatment of OSA in patients with CAD are less robust than for systemic hypertension.

A case-control study of 192 patients with acute MI (63 patients without OSA, 52 untreated patients with OSA, and 71 patients with OSA treated with CPAP), over a 6-year follow-up, showed that the risk of recurrent MI and revascularization procedures was lower in treated than in untreated OSA and was similar to patients without OSA.[126]

In another study, in 390 patients who had undergone percutaneous coronary intervention, over a median follow-up of 4.8 years, untreated OSA was independently associated with a significant increased risk of repeat revascularization that was reduced by CPAP treatment.[127]

SDB, in both forms of OSA and CSA, is common in patients with HF and has been suggested to increase the morbidity and mortality in these patients.

The mainstay of OSA treatment in HF is CPAP. Small studies showed that CPAP in patients with HF and OSA reduced 30-day hospital readmission and emergency visits.[128] It also improved systolic function, blood pressure, and heart rate.[129–131] In long-term studies, CPAP decreased mortality and improved hospitalization-free survival in patients with HF and OSA.[132,133] However, there are no double-blind randomized, controlled trials to evaluate these effects, particularly in the rehabilitation setting.

In contrast, studies in patients with HF and CSA suggested that CPAP also can improve EF[131,134] but does not show any survival benefit.[134] A recent randomized controlled trial (Adaptive Servo Ventilation in Patients with Heart Failure [SERVE-HF]) examined the effect of adaptive servoventilation in patients with reduced EF and CSA. This trial showed no significant positive effect, but increased both all-cause (HR, 1.28; 95% CI, 1.06–1.55; $P = .01$) and cardiovascular mortality (HR, 1.34; 95% CI, 1.09–1.65; $P = .006$).[135,136]

Therefore, until the results from further studies are available, optimization of HF management should be the first-line therapy in patients with concurrent CSA. Although the appropriate therapy for CSA in patients with HF remains controversial, CPAP remains widely accepted for OSA in patients with HF.

All of the studies discussed earlier show the beneficial effect of OSA treatment in the context of cardiac rehabilitation, and those patients should be screened early and considered for CPAP treatment until further robust clinical trials have been done.

SUMMARY

Several cohort studies have shown that OSA significantly increases the risk of cardiovascular disorders independently of potential confounding risk factors. This finding is particularly important given that sleep apnea is a potentially modifiable risk factor. Randomized controlled trials of CPAP in patients with OSA with follow-up of cerebrovascular and cardiovascular outcomes suggest a clinically significant risk reduction associated with the use of CPAP.

In view of potential benefits of noninvasive ventilation on prognosis and functional outcome with improving the quality of life, cognitive function, and acceleration of recovery in the rehabilitation of patients with cardiovascular diseases, clinicians should have a low threshold to evaluate their patients for SDB.

The reasons discussed earlier support the need for cardiac and stroke rehabilitation units to include sleep apnea screening and treatment as an integral component of their care.

REFERENCES

1. Young T, Palta M, Dempsey J, et al. The occurrence of sleep-disordered breathing among middle-aged adults. N Engl J Med 1993;328(17):1230–5.
2. Young T, Peppard PE, Gottlieb DJ. Epidemiology of obstructive sleep apnea: a population health perspective. Am J Respir Crit Care Med 2002; 165(9):1217–39.
3. Young TB. Epidemiology of daytime sleepiness: definitions, symptomatology, and prevalence. J Clin Psychiatry 2004;65(Suppl 16):12–6.
4. Sharma S, Parker AT. Prevalence of obstructive sleep apnea in a patient population undergoing cardiac rehabilitation. J Cardiopulm Rehabil Prev 2011;31(3):188–92.
5. Romero-Corral A, Somers VK, Pellikka PA, et al. Decreased right and left ventricular myocardial performance in obstructive sleep apnea. Chest 2007;132(6):1863–70.
6. Bonita R. Epidemiology of stroke. Lancet 1992; 339(8789):342–4.
7. Yaggi H, Mohsenin V. Obstructive sleep apnoea and stroke. Lancet Neurol 2004;3(6):333–42.
8. Cheyne JA. A case of apoplexy in which the fleshy part of the heart was converted into fat. Dublin Hosp Rep 1818;2:216–22.
9. Sahlin C, Sandberg O, Gustafson Y, et al. Obstructive sleep apnea is a risk factor for death in patients with stroke: a 10-year follow-up. Arch Intern Med 2008;168(3):297–301.
10. Kaneko Y, Hajek VE, Zivanovic V, et al. Relationship of sleep apnea to functional capacity and length of hospitalization following stroke. Sleep 2003;26: 293–7.
11. Brooks D, Davis L, Vujovic-Zotovic N, et al. Sleep-disordered breathing in patients enrolled in an inpatient stroke rehabilitation program. Arch Phys Med Rehabil 2010;91(4):659–62.
12. Bratton DJ, Gaisl T, Wons AM, et al. CPAP vs mandibular advancement devices and blood pressure in patients with obstructive sleep apnea: a systematic review and meta-analysis. JAMA 2015; 314:2280–93.
13. Ryan CM, Bayley M, Green R, et al. Influence of continuous positive airway pressure on outcomes of rehabilitation in stroke patients with obstructive sleep apnea. Stroke 2011;42(4):1062–7.
14. Sandberg O, Franklin KA, Bucht G, et al. Sleep apnea, delirium, depressed mood, cognition, and ADL ability after stroke. J Am Geriatr Soc 2001; 49(4):391–7.
15. Parra O, Sanchez-Armengol A, Bonnin M. Early treatment of obstructive sleep apnoea and stroke outcome: a randomised controlled trial. Eur Respir J 2011;011(37):1128–36.
16. Javaheri S. Sleep disorders in systolic heart failure: a prospective study of 100 male patients. The final report. Int J Cardiol 2006;106(1):21–8.
17. Bradley TD, Floras JS. Obstructive sleep apnoea and its cardiovascular consequences. Lancet 2009;373(9657):82–93.
18. Peppard PE, Young T, Palta M, et al. Prospective study of the association between sleep-disordered breathing and hypertension. N Engl J Med 2000; 342(19):1378–84.
19. Porthan KM, Melin JH, Kupila JT, et al. Prevalence of sleep apnea syndrome in lone atrial fibrillation: a case-control study. Chest 2004;125(3):879–85.
20. Young T, Peppard P, Palta M, et al. Population-based study of sleep-disordered breathing as a risk factor for hypertension. Arch Intern Med 1997;157(15):1746–52.
21. Nieto F, Young T, Lind B, et al. Association of sleep-disordered breathing, sleep apnea, and hypertension in a large community-based study. JAMA 2000;283:1229–36.
22. Hung J, Whitford EG, Parsons RW, et al. Association of sleep apnoea with myocardial infarction in men. Lancet 1990;336(8710):261–4.
23. Schafer H, Koehler U, Ewig S, et al. Obstructive sleep apnea as a risk marker in coronary artery disease. Cardiology 1999;92(2):79–84.
24. Cepeda-Valery B, Acharjee S, Romero-Corral A, et al. Obstructive sleep apnea and acute coronary syndromes: etiology, risk, and management. Curr Cardiol Rep 2014;16(10):535.
25. Khayat RN, Jarjoura D, Patt B, et al. In-hospital testing for sleep-disordered breathing in hospitalized patients with decompensated heart failure: report of prevalence and patient characteristics. J Card Fail 2009;15(9):739–46.
26. Oldenburg O, Lamp B, Faber L, et al. Sleep-disordered breathing in patients with symptomatic heart

failure: a contemporary study of prevalence in and characteristics of 700 patients. Eur J Heart Fail 2007;9(3):251–7.

27. Bitter T, Faber L, Hering D, et al. Sleep-disordered breathing in heart failure with normal left ventricular ejection fraction. Eur J Heart Fail 2009;11(6):602–8.

28. Buchner S, Satzl A, Debl K, et al. Impact of sleep-disordered breathing on myocardial salvage and infarct size in patients with acute myocardial infarction. Eur Heart J 2014;35(3):192–9.

29. Glantz H, Thunstrom E, Herlitz J, et al. Occurrence and predictors of obstructive sleep apnea in a revascularized coronary artery disease cohort. Ann Am Thorac Soc 2013;10(4):350–6.

30. Le Grande MR, Neubeck L, Murphy BM, et al. Screening for obstructive sleep apnoea in cardiac rehabilitation: a position statement from the Australian Centre for Heart Health and the Australian Cardiovascular Health and Rehabilitation Association. Eur J Prev Cardiol 2016;23(14):1466–75.

31. Bassetti C, Aldrich MS. Sleep apnea in acute cerebrovascular diseases: final report on 128 patients. Sleep 1999;22(2):217–23.

32. Bassetti C, Aldrich MS, Chervin RD, et al. Sleep apnea in patients with transient ischemic attack and stroke: a prospective study of 59 patients. Neurology 1996;47(5):1167–73.

33. Bassetti C, Aldrich MS, Quint D. Sleep-disordered breathing in patients with acute supra- and infra-tentorial strokes. A prospective study of 39 patients. Stroke 1997;28(9):1765–72.

34. Parra O, Arboix A, Bechich S, et al. Time course of sleep-related breathing disorders in first-ever stroke or transient ischemic attack. Am J Respir Crit Care Med 2000;161(2 Pt 1):375–80.

35. Arzt M, Young T, Finn L, et al. Association of sleep-disordered breathing and the occurrence of stroke. Am J Respir Crit Care Med 2005;172(11):1447–51.

36. Dyken ME, Somers VK, Yamada T, et al. Investigating the relationship between stroke and obstructive sleep apnea. Stroke 1996;27(3):401–7.

37. Good DC, Henkle JQ, Gelber D, et al. Sleep-disordered breathing and poor functional outcome after stroke. Stroke 1996;27(2):252–9.

38. Parra O. Sleep-disordered breathing and stroke: is there a rationale for treatment? Eur Respir J 2001; 18(4):619–22.

39. Broadley SA, Jorgensen L, Cheek A, et al. Early investigation and treatment of obstructive sleep apnoea after acute stroke. J Clin Neurosci 2007; 14(4):328–33.

40. Mohsenin V, Valor R. Sleep apnea in patients with hemispheric stroke. Arch Phys Med Rehabil 1995; 76(1):71–6.

41. Yaggi H, Concato J, Kernan W, et al. Obstructive sleep apnea as a risk factor for stroke and death. N Engl J Med 2005;353:2034–41.

42. Munoz R, Duran-Cantolla J, Martinez-Vila E, et al. Severe sleep apnea and risk of ischemic stroke in the elderly. Stroke 2006;37(9):2317–21.

43. Young T, Finn L, Peppard PE, et al. Sleep disordered breathing and mortality: eighteen-year follow-up of the Wisconsin sleep cohort. Sleep 2008;31(8):1071–8.

44. Marin JM, Carrizo SJ, Vicente E, et al. Long-term cardiovascular outcomes in men with obstructive sleep apnoea-hypopnoea with or without treatment with continuous positive airway pressure: an observational study. Lancet 2005;365(9464):1046–53.

45. Lai SM, Studenski S, Duncan PW, et al. Persisting consequences of stroke measured by the Stroke Impact Scale. Stroke 2002;33(7):1840–4.

46. Dziewas R, Humpert M, Hopmann B, et al. Increased prevalence of sleep apnea in patients with recurring ischemic stroke compared with first stroke victims. J Neurol 2005;252(11):1394–8.

47. Bravata DM, Concato J, Fried T, et al. Continuous positive airway pressure: evaluation of a novel therapy for patients with acute ischemic stroke. Sleep 2011;34(9):1271–7.

48. Szücs A, Vitrai J, Janszky J, et al. Pathological sleep apnoea frequency remains permanent in ischaemic stroke and it is transient in haemorrhagic stroke. Eur Neurol 2002;47(1):15–9.

49. Tosun A, Kokturk O, Karata GK, et al. Obstructive sleep apnea in ischemic stroke patients. Clinics (Sao Paulo) 2008;63(5):625–30.

50. Hermann DM, Siccoli M, Kirov P, et al. Central periodic breathing during sleep in acute ischemic stroke. Stroke 2007;38(3):1082–4.

51. Rola R, Wierzbicka A, Wichniak A, et al. Sleep related breathing disorders in patients with ischemic stroke and transient ischemic attacks: respiratory and clinical correlations. J Physiol Pharmacol 2007;58 Suppl 5(Pt 2):575–82.

52. Rowat AM, Dennis MS, Wardlaw JM. Central periodic breathing observed on hospital admission is associated with an adverse prognosis in conscious acute stroke patients. Cerebrovasc Dis 2006;21(5–6):340–7.

53. Bassetti CL, Milanova M, Gugger M. Sleep-disordered breathing and acute ischemic stroke: diagnosis, risk factors, treatment, evolution, and long-term clinical outcome. Stroke 2006;37(4):967–72.

54. Arzt M, Young T, Peppard PE, et al. Dissociation of obstructive sleep apnea from hypersomnolence and obesity in patients with stroke. Stroke 2010; 41(3):e129–34.

55. Bennett LS, Stradling JR, Davies RJ. A behavioural test to assess daytime sleepiness in obstructive sleep apnoea. J Sleep Res 1997;6(2):142–5.

56. Wessendorf TE, Wang YM, Thilmann AF, et al. Treatment of obstructive sleep apnoea with nasal

continuous positive airway pressure in stroke. Eur Respir J 2001;18(4):623–9.

57. Punjabi NM, Bandeen-Roche K, Young T. Predictors of objective sleep tendency in the general population. Sleep 2003;26(6):678–83.

58. Javaheri S, Parker TJ, Liming JD, et al. Sleep apnea in 81 ambulatory male patients with stable heart failure. Types and their prevalences, consequences, and presentations. Circulation 1998; 97(21):2154–9.

59. Arzt M, Young T, Finn L, et al. Sleepiness and sleep in patients with both systolic heart failure and obstructive sleep apnea. Arch Intern Med 2006; 166(16):1716–22.

60. Kryger M, Roth T, Dement WC, editors. Principles and practice of sleep medicine. 4th edition. Philadelphia: Elsevier Saunders; 2005.

61. Duran J, Esnaola S, Rubio R, et al. Obstructive sleep apnea-hypopnea and related clinical features in a population-based sample of subjects aged 30 to 70 yr. Am J Respir Crit Care Med 2001;163(3 Pt 1):685–9.

62. Young T, Shahar E, Nieto FJ, et al. Predictors of sleep-disordered breathing in community-dwelling adults: the Sleep Heart Health Study. Arch Intern Med 2002;162(8):893–900.

63. Gottlieb DJ, Whitney CW, Bonekat WH, et al. Relation of sleepiness to respiratory disturbance index: the Sleep Heart Health Study. Am J Respir Crit Care Med 1999;159(2):502–7.

64. Banack HR, Holly CD, Lowensteyn I, et al. The association between sleep disturbance, depressive symptoms, and health-related quality of life among cardiac rehabilitation participants. J cardiopulmonary Rehabil Prev 2014;34(3):188–94.

65. Redeker NS, Ruggiero J, Hedges C. Patterns and predictors of sleep pattern disturbance after cardiac surgery. Res Nurs Health 2004;27(4):217–24.

66. Hargens TA, Aron A, Newsome LJ, et al. Effects of obstructive sleep apnea on hemodynamic parameters in patients entering cardiac rehabilitation. J cardiopulmonary Rehabil Prev 2015;35(3):181–5.

67. Uchoa CH, Danzi-Soares Nde J, Nunes FS, et al. Impact of OSA on cardiovascular events after coronary artery bypass surgery. Chest 2015;147(5): 1352–60.

68. Decary A, Rouleau I, Montplaisir J. Cognitive deficits associated with sleep apnea syndrome: a proposed neuropsychological test battery. Sleep 2000;23(3):369–81.

69. Sandberg O, Franklin KA, Bucht G, et al. Nasal continuous positive airway pressure in stroke patients with sleep apnoea: a randomized treatment study. Eur Respir J 2001;18(4):630–4.

70. Harbison J, Ford GA, James OF, et al. Sleep-disordered breathing following acute stroke. QJM 2002; 95(11):741–7.

71. Iranzo A, Santamaria J, Berenguer J, et al. Prevalence and clinical importance of sleep apnea in the first night after cerebral infarction. Neurology 2002;58(6):911–6.

72. Turkington PM. Effect of upper airway obstruction on blood pressure variability after stroke [comment]. Clin Sci 2004;107(1):27–8.

73. Gami AS, Howard DE, Olson EJ, et al. Day-night pattern of sudden death in obstructive sleep apnea. N Engl J Med 2005;352(12):1206–14.

74. Martinez-Garcia MA, Soler-Cataluna JJ, Ejarque-Martinez L, et al. Continuous positive airway pressure treatment reduces mortality in patients with ischemic stroke and obstructive sleep apnea: a 5-year follow-up study. Am J Respir Crit Care Med 2009;180(1):36–41.

75. Parra O, Arboix A, Montserrat JM, et al. Sleep-related breathing disorders: impact on mortality of cerebrovascular disease. Eur Respir J 2004; 24(2):267–72.

76. Turkington PM, Bamford J, Wanklyn P, et al. Effect of upper airway obstruction on blood pressure variability after stroke. Clin Sci (Lond) 2004; 107(1):75–9.

77. Balfors EM, Franklin KA. Impairment of cerebral perfusion during obstructive sleep apneas. Am J Respir Crit Care Med 1994;150(6 Pt 1):1587–91.

78. Alessi CA, Martin JL, Webber AP, et al. More daytime sleeping predicts less functional recovery among older people undergoing inpatient post-acute rehabilitation. Sleep 2008;31(9):1291–300.

79. Barbar SI, Enright PL, Boyle P, et al. Sleep disturbances and their correlates in elderly Japanese American men residing in Hawaii. J Gerontol A Biol Sci Med Sci 2000;55(7):M406–11.

80. Kutner NG, Schechtman KB, Ory MG, et al. Older adults' perceptions of their health and functioning in relation to sleep disturbance, falling, and urinary incontinence. FICSIT Group. J Am Geriatr Soc 1994;42(7):757–62.

81. Schmitt FA, Phillips BA, Cook YR, et al. Self report on sleep symptoms in older adults: correlates of daytime sleepiness and health. Sleep 1996;19(1): 59–64.

82. Alessi CA, Martin JL, Webber AP, et al. Randomized, controlled trial of a nonpharmacological intervention to improve abnormal sleep/wake patterns in nursing home residents. J Am Geriatr Soc 2005;53(5):803–10.

83. Martin JL, Webber AP, Alam T, et al. Daytime sleeping, sleep disturbance, and circadian rhythms in the nursing home. Am J Geriatr Psychiatry 2006;14(2):121–9.

84. Ohayon MM, Vecchierini MF. Normative sleep data, cognitive function and daily living activities in older adults in the community. Sleep 2005; 28(8):981–9.

85. Wessendorf TE, Teschler H, Wang YM, et al. Sleep-disordered breathing among patients with first-ever stroke. J Neurol 2000;247(1):41–7.

86. Hoogerduijn JG, Schuurmans MJ, Duijnstee MS, et al. A systematic review of predictors and screening instruments to identify older hospitalized patients at risk for functional decline. J Clin Nurs 2007;16(1):46–57.

87. Hayano J, Carney RM, Watanabe E, et al. Interactive associations of depression and sleep apnea with adverse clinical outcomes after acute myocardial infarction. Psychosom Med 2012;74(8):832–9.

88. Le Grande MR, Jackson AC, Murphy BM, et al. Relationship between sleep disturbance, depression and anxiety in the 12 months following a cardiac event. Psychol Health Med 2016;21(1):52–9.

89. Hamilton BB, Granger CV, Sherwin FS, et al. A uniform national data system for medical rehabilitation. In: Fuhrer M, editor. Rehabilitation outcomes: analysis and measurement. Baltimore (MD): Brookes; 1987. p. 137–47.

90. Granger CV, Cotter AC, Hamilton BB, et al. Functional assessment scales: a study of persons after stroke. Arch Phys Med Rehabil 1993;74(2):133–8.

91. Turkington PM, Allgar V, Bamford J, et al. Effect of upper airway obstruction in acute stroke on functional outcome at 6 months. Thorax 2004;59(5):367–71.

92. Kales A, Caldwell AB, Cadieux RJ, et al. Severe obstructive sleep apnea–II: associated psychopathology and psychosocial consequences. J Chronic Dis 1985;38(5):427–34.

93. Leegaard OF. Diffuse cerebral symptoms in convalescents from cerebral infarction and myocardial infarction. Acta Neurol Scand 1983;67(6):348–55.

94. Siddiqui F, Macrea M, Horowitz M, et al. Relationship between excessive daytime sleepiness and 6 minute walk test in patients with coronary artery disease and obstructive sleep apnea. Chest 2015;148:1064A.

95. Leppavuori A, Pohjasvaara T, Vataja R, et al. Insomnia in ischemic stroke patients. Cerebrovasc Dis 2002;14(2):90–7.

96. Gustafson Y, Nilsson I, Mattsson M, et al. Epidemiology and treatment of post-stroke depression. Drugs Aging 1995;7(4):298–309.

97. Foley DJ, Monjan AA, Brown SL, et al. Sleep complaints among elderly persons: an epidemiologic study of three communities. Sleep 1995;18(6):425–32.

98. Findley LJ, Barth JT, Powers DC, et al. Cognitive impairment in patients with obstructive sleep apnea and associated hypoxemia. Chest 1986;90(5):686–90.

99. Millman RP, Fogel BS, McNamara ME, et al. Depression as a manifestation of obstructive sleep apnea: reversal with nasal continuous positive airway pressure. J Clin Psychiatry 1989;50(9):348–51.

100. Montplaisir J, Bedard MA, Richer F, et al. Neurobehavioral manifestations in obstructive sleep apnea syndrome before and after treatment with continuous positive airway pressure. Sleep 1992;15(6 Suppl):S17–9.

101. Vgontzas AN, Liao D, Bixler EO, et al. Insomnia with objective short sleep duration is associated with a high risk for hypertension. Sleep 2009;32(4):491–7.

102. Langhorne P, Stott DJ, Robertson L, et al. Medical complications after stroke: a multicenter study. Stroke 2000;31(6):1223–9.

103. McManus J, Pathansali R, Hassan H, et al. The course of delirium in acute stroke. Age Ageing 2009;38(4):385–9.

104. McManus J, Pathansali R, Stewart R, et al. Delirium post-stroke. Age Ageing 2007;36(6):613–8.

105. Gustafson Y, Olsson T, Eriksson S, et al. Acute confusional states in stroke patients. Cerebrovasc Dis 1991;1:257–64.

106. Whitney JF, Gannon DE. Obstructive sleep apnea presenting as acute delirium. Am J Emerg Med 1996;14(3):270–1.

107. Lee JW. Recurrent delirium associated with obstructive sleep apnea. Gen Hosp Psychiatry 1998;20(2):120–2.

108. Munoz X, Marti S, Sumalla J, et al. Acute delirium as a manifestation of obstructive sleep apnea syndrome. Am J Respir Crit Care Med 1998;158(4):1306–7.

109. Minnerup J, Ritter MA, Wersching H, et al. Continuous positive airway pressure ventilation for acute ischemic stroke. A randomized feasibility study. Stroke 2012;43:1137–9.

110. Becker H, Jerrentrup A, Ploch T, et al. Effect of nasal continuous positive airway pressure treatment on blood pressure in patients with obstructive sleep apnea. Circulation 2003;107:68–73.

111. Martinez-Garcia MA, Galiano-Blancart R, Roman-Sanchez P, et al. Continuous positive airway pressure treatment in sleep apnea prevents new vascular events after ischemic stroke. Chest 2005;128(4):2123–9.

112. Bravata DM, Concato J, Fried T, et al. Auto-titrating continuous positive airway pressure for patients with acute transient ischemic attack: a randomized feasibility trial. Stroke 2010;41(7):1464–70.

113. Hui DS, Choy DK, Wong LK, et al. Prevalence of sleep-disordered breathing and continuous positive airway pressure compliance: results in Chinese patients with first-ever ischemic stroke. Chest 2002;122(3):852–60.

114. Hsu CY, Vennelle M, Li HY, et al. Sleep-disordered breathing after stroke: a randomised controlled trial

of continuous positive airway pressure. J Neurol Neurosurg Psychiatry 2006;77(10):1143–9.

115. Brown DL, Chervin RD, Kalbfleisch JD, et al. Sleep Apnea Treatment After Stroke (SATS) trial: is it feasible? J Stroke Cerebrovas Dis 2013;22(8): 1216–24.

116. Palombini L, Guilleminault C. Stroke and treatment with nasal CPAP. Eur J Neurol 2006;13(2):198–200.

117. Scala R, Turkington PM, Wanklyn P, et al. Acceptance, effectiveness and safety of continuous positive airway pressure in acute stroke: a pilot study. Respir Med 2009;103(1):59–66.

118. Partinen M, Guilleminault C. Daytime sleepiness and vascular morbidity at seven-year follow-up in obstructive sleep apnea patients. Chest 1990; 97(1):27–32.

119. Marti S, Sampol G, Munoz X, et al. Mortality in severe sleep apnoea/hypopnoea syndrome patients: impact of treatment. Eur Respir J 2002; 20(6):1511–8.

120. Doherty L, Kiely J, Swan V, et al. Long-term effects of nasal continuous positive airways pressure therapy on cardiovascular outcomes in sleep apnea syndrome. Chest 2005;127(6):2076–84.

121. Faccenda J, Mackay T, Boon N, et al. Randomized placebo-controlled trial of continuous positive airway pressure on blood pressure in the sleep apnea-hypopnea syndrome. Am J Respir Crit Care Med 2001;163:344–8.

122. Pepperell JC, Ramdassingh-Dow S, Crosthwaite N, et al. Ambulatory blood pressure after therapeutic and subtherapeutic nasal continuous positive airway pressure for obstructive sleep apnoea: a randomised parallel trial. Lancet 2002;359(9302): 204–10.

123. Barbe F, Mayoralas LR, Duran J, et al. Treatment with continuous positive airway pressure is not effective in patients with sleep apnea but no daytime sleepiness. a randomized, controlled trial. Ann Intern Med 2001;134(11):1015–23.

124. Monasterio C, Vidal S, Duran J, et al. Effectiveness of continuous positive airway pressure in mild sleep apnea-hypopnea syndrome. Am J Respir Crit Care Med 2001;164(6):939–43.

125. Collins R, Peto R, MacMahon S, et al. Blood pressure, stroke, and coronary heart disease. Part 2, short-term reductions in blood pressure: overview of randomised drug trials in their epidemiological context. Lancet 1990;335(8693):827–38.

126. Garcia-Rio F, Alonso-Fernandez A, Armada E, et al. CPAP effect on recurrent episodes in patients with sleep apnea and myocardial infarction. Int J Cardiol 2013;168(2):1328–35.

127. Wu X, Lv S, Yu X, et al. Treatment of OSA reduces the risk of repeat revascularization after percutaneous coronary intervention. Chest 2015;147(3): 708–18.

128. Kauta SR, Keenan BT, Goldberg L, et al. Diagnosis and treatment of sleep disordered breathing in hospitalized cardiac patients: a reduction in 30-day hospital readmission rates. J Clin Sleep Med 2014;10(10):1051–9.

129. Kaneko Y, Floras JS, Usui K, et al. Cardiovascular effects of continuous positive airway pressure in patients with heart failure and obstructive sleep apnea. N Engl J Med 2003;348(13):1233–41.

130. Mansfield DR, Gollogly NC, Kaye DM, et al. Controlled trial of continuous positive airway pressure in obstructive sleep apnea and heart failure. Am J Respir Crit Care Med 2004;169(3):361–6.

131. Sun H, Shi J, Li M, et al. Impact of continuous positive airway pressure treatment on left ventricular ejection fraction in patients with obstructive sleep apnea: a meta-analysis of randomized controlled trials. PLoS One 2013;8(5):e62298.

132. Wang H, Parker JD, Newton GE, et al. Influence of obstructive sleep apnea on mortality in patients with heart failure. J Am Coll Cardiol 2007;49(15): 1625–31.

133. Kasai T, Narui K, Dohi T, et al. Prognosis of patients with heart failure and obstructive sleep apnea treated with continuous positive airway pressure. Chest 2008;133(3):690–6.

134. Bradley TD, Logan AG, Kimoff RJ, et al. Continuous positive airway pressure for central sleep apnea and heart failure. N Engl J Med 2005;353(19): 2025–33.

135. Cowie MR, Wegscheider K, Teschler H. Adaptive servo-ventilation for central sleep apnea in heart failure. N Engl J Med 2016;374(7):690–1.

136. Cowie MR, Woehrle H, Wegscheider K, et al. Adaptive servo-ventilation for central sleep apnea in systolic heart failure. N Engl J Med 2015;373(12): 1095–105.

A Practical Approach to the Identification and Management of Sleep-Disordered Breathing in Heart Failure Patients

Rami Kahwash, MD[a],*, Rami N. Khayat, MD[b]

KEYWORDS

- Sleep apnea • Obstructive • Central • Heart failure • Chronic • Systolic • Respiration
- Positive airway pressure

KEY POINTS

- Sleep-disordered breathing remains a prevalent comorbidity in patients with heart failure and is associated with poor outcome.
- Screening for sleep-disordered breathing should be performed routinely among heart failure patients because of high prevalence and etiologic association with many risk factors.
- Lifestyle modifications, restoring euvolemic state, and optimizing heart failure medical and device-based therapies are essential steps in the treatment of sleep-disordered breathing in heart failure patients.
- Treatment of obstructive sleep apnea in heart failure with continuous positive airway pressure was not associated with reduction in mortality or cardiovascular end points in a recent large randomized trial.
- Continuous positive airway pressure therapy should continue to be considered in heart failure patients with obstructive sleep apnea based on sufficient evidence for safety and effect on sleep quality and daytime function.
- There is no clinical evidence thus far to suggest any effective therapeutic option for central sleep apnea among heart failure patients. Although the roles of pressure support therapies for central sleep apnea in heart failure still require further investigation, an implantable phrenic nerve stimulator may offer a promising therapeutic option.

INTRODUCTION

Sleep-disordered breathing (SDB) is prevalent in patients with both systolic and diastolic heart failure (HF), representing the most common comorbidity and affecting between 50% and 80% of all patients.[1–3] SDB is classified further into obstructive sleep apnea (OSA), which is caused by intermittent obstruction in the upper airways, and central sleep apnea (CSA), which is defined as a periodic loss of central respiratory drive. Both OSA and CSA share a common pattern of

The authors have no relevant conflicts of interest.
[a] Section of Heart Failure and Transplant, Division of Cardiovascular Medicine, Davis Heart & Lung Research Institute, The Ohio State University, 473 West 12th Avenue, Columbus, OH 43210, USA; [b] Division of Pulmonary, Allergy, Critical Care, and Sleep Medicine, Davis Heart & Lung Research Institute, The Ohio State University, 473 West 12th Avenue, Columbus, OH 43210, USA
* Corresponding author.
E-mail address: Rami.Kahwash@osumc.edu

Sleep Med Clin 12 (2017) 205–219
http://dx.doi.org/10.1016/j.jsmc.2017.01.002
1556-407X/17/© 2017 Elsevier Inc. All rights reserved.

repetitive hypoxemia and arousals resulting in sympathetic activation, oxidative stress, and sleep disruption. Therefore, both types of SDB have a negative impact on quality of life and cardiovascular function. It is well known that SDB treatment improves markers of cardiovascular disease and lessens their progression into HF. Furthermore, among HF patients, untreated SDB is independently linked to worse outcome. Although treatment of SDB is safe, readily available, and associated with improvement in cardiac function and quality of life of HF patients, data on improving outcomes are disappointing thus far. Despite the high prevalence of SDB in HF patients, the sleep and HF organizations have not provided treating physicians with practice guidelines to advise management of SDB in HF patients. This lack of guidelines has created large deviations in practice standards and explains why only a small fraction of HF patients receive adequate screening and treatment of SDB.[4]

This article provides a comprehensive overview of SDB in HF with focus on practical screening algorithms and simplified therapeutic approaches to help clinicians better recognize and treat SDB among their HF patients.

DEFINITION AND CLASSIFICATION OF SLEEP-DISORDERED BREATHING

SDB encompasses breathing irregularities that mainly take place during sleep. They are characterized by cyclic pauses of sleep with ensuing hypoxia followed by partial neurologic arousals. This frequent disruption in sleep architecture produces several deleterious neurohormonal and oxidative effects that extend beyond sleep hours to the waking time.

SDB events are classified into apneas and hypopneas. Apnea is a complete cessation of breathing and is further classified into obstructive or central based on the presence or absence of associated effort. Hypopneas are episodes of decreased air flow and are often difficult to further classify into obstructive or central. SDB is generally classified into OSA and CSA based on the dominant type of events. In other words, if more than half of the events were classified as obstructive, the SDB is classified as OSA. Similarly, CSA is diagnosed when more than half of the events are classified as central. In both OSA and CSA, the severity of SDB is judged by the Apnea Hypopnea Index (AHI), which reflects the number of apnea or hypopnea episodes per hour of sleep. Mild disease is defined as an AHI of 5 to 15 per hour, moderate as 15 to 30 per hour, and severe as ≥30 per hour. OSA is common in the general population

and in HF compared with CSA, which is mainly found in advanced HF. Importantly, it is well established that patients with HF can shift between one type of SDB to another from night to night.[5] The coexistence of OSA and CSA in the same HF patient can also manifest in having high percentage of central events in a patient classified as having OSA. The prevalence of these mixed SDB cases among HF patients is not reported. In the HF population, it is not uncommon to see both types of SDB coexist in the same patient.

THE EPIDEMIOLOGY OF SLEEP-DISORDERED BREATHING IN HEART FAILURE

SDB is prevalent in the overall population and more so in patients with HF. In the general public, the incidence of SDB among middle-age adults is estimated to be 9% to 24%,[6] whereas patients with AHI of ≥5 accounted for more 24% among the elderly in one study.[7]

In patients with HF, the prevalence of SDB far exceeds that of the general population.[1,6,8] Earlier epidemiologic studies estimated a prevalence of 24% to 37% for OSA and 40% for CSA in patients with HF.[1,6,8] Other reports showed higher prevalence of OSA than CSA in patients with chronic HF.[9,10] Studies of hospitalized patients with acute decompensated heart failure confirmed a higher prevalence of OSA in the inpatient population.[11] This finding could be explained by the strong association of OSA and cardiovascular risk factors that manifest clinically during the decompensated state.[12–14] Additionally, the increasing incidence of obesity in the general population, and the relation between obesity, OSA, and cardiovascular disease, lends further explanation to the higher prevalence of OSA among HF patients. CSA, however, is considered mainly a disorder of advanced stages of systolic HF and its relationship to common cardiac risk factors is not as strong as that of OSA.[1,11]

The prevalence of OSA in diastolic HF is less studied than it is in systolic HF. However, SDB seem to affect both types of HF at a similar rate. In one report, AHI of 10 or more was present in 50% of patients with isolated diastolic HF.[15]

There is also significant sex variation in the occurrence of SDB with men being more affected than women. The exact reason for sex mismatch is still unclear but can be attributed to the android pattern of weight gain seen in men and also to the effects of testosterone on respiratory centers and upper airway musculature.[16]

Age is a major risk factor for OSA in the middle-age population. After the age of 60, sex and weight become less important predictors of OSA; this is possibly because of the predominant effect of aging on the upper airway tone, which weakens the impact of the other risk factors.[17]

PATHOPHYSIOLOGY OF SLEEP DISORDERED BREATHING
Obstructive Sleep Apnea

OSA is very prevalent and affects more than 20% of the general population and at least 35% of patients with HF.[3,4] OSA is characterized by partial or complete upper airway obstruction during sleep caused by a reduced or loss of pharyngeal dilator tone resulting in cessation of the airflow despite continued respiratory effort of the thoracic and abdominal muscles. The upper airway obstruction and associated hypoxia continues until awakening when airway patency is restored. The recurrence of these respiratory events results in cyclic nocturnal intermittent hypoxia and frequent neurologic arousals, which impact quality of life and reduce daytime energy level. Each episode of hypoxia triggers sympathetic nerve activation[18] with subsequent surge in pulmonary and systemic vasoconstriction.[19]

Unlike other forms of hypoxia, intermittent nocturnal hypoxia is a distinct physiologic state that is stressful to the cardiopulmonary and cardiovascular systems with significant deleterious biological consequences.[20–23] Intermittent hypoxia has been shown in animal and human models to cause daytime hypertension[24–26] and is an independent risk factor for hypertension[27] and ischemic heart disease.[28,29]

The etiologic relationship between OSA and other HF risks factors, including coronary artery disease,[30,31] hypertension, and arrhythmia,[32,33] distinguishes OSA as an independent risk factor for HF development.[34] Furthermore, those deleterious effects on cardiovascular function and cardiopulmonary hemodynamics are more pronounced in the HF state.

OSA also creates hemodynamic changes that negatively impact cardiac performance and cardiac output. During an OSA event, the continuous respiratory effort against an occluded pharynx causes tremendous increase in the negative intrathoracic pressure. This process further leads to an increase in left ventricular transmural gradient, which is determined by the difference between intrathoracic and intracranial pressures. Such changes accentuate left ventricular wall tension, with consequent increases in afterload and decreases in cardiac output.[35]

The hemodynamic effects of OSA are not restricted to the left ventricle only; they extend to disturb the right ventricular function and interventricular dynamics. Negative intrathoracic pressure that occurs during an OSA event enhances venous return to the right ventricle and causes an increase in right ventricular preload. Overfilling of the right ventricle mechanically shifts the intraventricular septum toward the left ventricle, which decreases the left ventricular end-diastolic volume with an ensuing drop in preload.[36] As a result, OSA mediated by increasing afterload and decreasing preload reduces cardiac output and alters cardiopulmonary hemodynamics in a way that leads to ineffective circulation.

Heart rate tends to be elevated in patients with OSA, as repetitive obstructive cycles and heightened sympathetic activation prevent the normal dipping in nocturnal heart rate seen in normal physiologic state. Elevation in heart rate and blood pressure[27] leads to a higher myocardial metabolic requirement, which predisposes patients to supply-demand ischemia, myocyte irritability, and lethal arrhythmias.[37] Altered hemodynamics and activation of neurohormonal accesses intensify systemic inflammatory response. Inflammatory markers, manifested by the level of C-reactive protein levels, increased in SDB and correlated well with the severity of AHI in patients with OSA.[38]

OSA is associated with abnormal hemodynamic and vascular effects that are the sequelae of OSA-induced alterations in intrathoracic pressures and activation of the sympathetic nervous system, which predispose to the development of hypertension, myocardial ischemia, and arrhythmias and eventually lead to worsening left ventricular function and rapid progression to clinical HF. This finding was confirmed in a large respective, longitudinal epidemiologic study that established the link between OSA and increasing occurrence of HF in middle-age and older men.[39]

Central Sleep Apnea

Although CSA is rarely seen in the general population, it is very common in HF patients irrespective of the left ventricular function. In HF with reduced ejection fraction, CSA is estimated to affect 30% to 50% of the total patients.[3,40–42] Its prevalence, however, is lower in HF with preserved ejection fraction, where it affects 18% to 13% of all patients.[15,43,44]

In CSA, the respiratory disturbances are characterized by recurrent cycles of temporary loss of central respiratory output, causing absence of respiratory muscle movements followed by loss of upper airway flow and arterial oxygen desaturation.[45–47] Cheyne-Stokes respiration is a distinct type of CSA seen in HF and characterized by absence of chest wall movements accompanied by loss of upper airway flow and oxygen desaturation, followed by up and down fluctuations in the frequency and depth of the breathing cycles in a crescendo-decrescendo pattern. Clinically, it manifests as periods of hypoventilation and apnea alternating with cycles of hyperventilation.

In normal state, spontaneous respiration is meticulously regulated by partial pressure of carbon dioxide, arterial ($Paco_2$) level through its effect on central chemoreceptors, which regulate respiratory drive and effort to keep $Paco_2$ in the normal range. In HF patients, this regulatory feedback mechanism is impaired. Pulmonary congestion, which is commonly seen in HF, causes distension and stimulation of the stretch receptors in lung vessels, which subsequently leads to excessive ventilation and chronic hypocapnia.[48] In this chronic hypocapnic state, $Paco_2$ periodically decreases to below the apnea threshold causing abrupt loss of respiratory drive, followed by immediate increase in $Paco_2$ level and sudden arousal from sleep.[8,45] Hypoxia, which also occurs during the central apneic episode, further contributes to neurologic arousal and hyperventilation response. Once hyperventilation occurs, $Paco_2$ gradually declines until it decreases to below the apnea threshold, and a new cycle starts again.

Although fluctuation of $Paco_2$ greater than and less than the apnea threshold is believed to be the main mechanism in CSA, other factors may be contributing as well. Upper airway instability, diminished cerebrovascular response to changes in $Paco_2$ levels, low cardiac output with resultant prolonged circulation, and mismatch between central and peripheral chemoreceptor responses, all contribute to the perpetuation of CSA cyclic events.[49–52]

Similar to OSA, recurrent cycles of apnea and hyperventilation in CSA incite deleterious hemodynamic and neurohormonal changes including tachycardia, systemic vasoconstriction, sodium retention, and rennin angiotensin system activation that are deleterious to the failing heart.[53,54] Activation of the sympathetic system in CSA also leads to an increase in ventricular irritability, which can be lowered by treating CSA.[55,56] Additionally, data showed close association between CSA and atrial fibrillation.[40]

Arousal from sleep is associated with rapid increase in heart rate and blood pressure[8,57] and may also prompt the induction of lethal arrhythmias.[8,58] CSA is a known independent risk factor in HF, and its presence is linked to worse prognosis,[59] including hospital admission, cardiac transplantation, and death.[56,60,61] This worse prognosis is believed to be in part mediated by the cardiotoxic effect of catecholamines, which are found in higher concentrations in the urine of patients with advanced HF and CSA compared with those without CSA.[62]

Recognition of Sleep-Disordered Breathing in Heart Failure

SDB is the most prevalent comorbidity the HF populations and is associated with increased morbidity and mortality. Despite that finding, only a small fraction of HF patients receives adequate screening and treatment, in part because of the lack of commonly adopted surveillance strategy among medical care providers. Having a high index of suspicion and implementing systemic methods in identifying patients at risk of SDB among HF patients are perhaps the most vital steps in the management. Recognition of SDB is a multileveled process that starts with taking comprehensive sleep history and performing focused physical examination and concludes with referring high-risk patients for specific sleep testing and specialized sleep clinics, when indicated.

Comprehensive heart sleep history

A sleep history should be obtained in all HF patients as part of their initial evaluation. Symptoms of SDB include habitual snoring, witnessed apnea, excessive daytime sleepiness, excessive fatigue, lethargy, diminished concentration, impaired memory, and paroxysmal nocturnal dyspnea. Most of these symptoms could be attributed to frequent interruptions in the sleep cycle and deprivation from reaching deep sleep stages. Although none of these symptoms has been proven to solely predict SDB in HF, patients with HF tend to have at least one or more of those signs that warrant further screening. Because these symptoms are commonly seen in HF, SDB is often missed or unrecognized during routine HF evaluation. Additionally, the side effects of HF medications, such as β-blockers (BB), include excessive lethargy, which may divert attention from SDB. Screening for SDB should not be restricted to the outpatient setting in HF. In fact, hospitalized patients with acute decompensated HF may manifest the signs and symptoms of SDB more prominently as congestion and volume overload perpetuate many of SDB features. The inpatient setting provides an ideal environment to screen for SDB, as it allows close monitoring of patients' sleeping pattern, oxygenation, and changes in hemodynamics.[11]

Several patient-based questionnaires were developed to aid in SDB screening, such as Epworth Sleeping Scale[63,64] and Berlin

Questionnaire.[65] Although those questionnaires were proven effective in the general population, they did not add diagnostic value in the HF population.[66] Therefore, when questionnaires determine there is no HF, further evaluation of SDB should not be withheld, especially if clinical suspicion is high. Because of the high prevalence of SDB in HF and availably of effective therapies, a low of index of suspicion must be maintained in all HF patients.[11]

Clinical examination in sleep-disordered breathing

Careful physical examination is a fundamental step in screening for SDB. The examiner should focus on the presence of known high-risk features such as male sex, older age, obesity, and history of snoring. Obesity in most individuals is associated with anatomic changes in the neck related to excessive adipose tissue deposit, which contributes to pharyngeal obstruction.[67] Obesity's effect on SDB is not universal throughout age groups and tend to be less important in patients older than 60 years because of the predominate effect of reduced pharyngeal dilators seen in the elderly.[17]

The presentation of OSA, in particular, is less affected by obesity in HF patients compared with those without HF.[66] In nonobese HF patients, it seems like the central and cranial fluid shifts that happen in supine positions are major contributors to the increase in neck congestion, which leads to pharyngeal edema and upper airway obstruction.[68,69]

Findings that suggest increased risks of SDB on physical examination include crowded pharynx, redundant tissue and elongated soft palate, small jaw, and engorged uvula.[67] The Mallampati airway classification is commonly used to assess the severity of upper way obstruction and risks of OSA. It has been validated in the general population, but data on its usefulness in HF are lacking.[70]

Screening for CSA by clinical assessment is much more difficult than that for OSA, as CSA patients are not overweight in general and tend not to snore as often.[1] Because CSA occurs more frequently in patients with advanced HF stages, clinical signs of severe HF should raise the suspicion of CSA, including diminished functional class, depressed left ventricular ejection fraction, chronic hypocapnia, presence of atrial fibrillation, higher brain natriuretic peptide levels, and frequent nocturnal ventricular arrhythmias.[1,41,42,71]

Sleep-disordered breathing testing

If clinical history and physical examination are highly suggestive of SDB, the next step should be referring patients to specific sleep testing designed to confirm the diagnosis and assess the type and severity of SDB. Nocturnal polysomnography (NPSG) performed in designated sleep laboratories is the gold standard in SDB evaluation; however, this test has many limitations. Thus, simpler portable sleep monitors used by patients in the convenience of their homes have recently become more significant.

Nocturnal polysomnography NPSG is the gold standard test for the diagnosis SDB. It involves an overnight stay at a sleep laboratory, during which sleep and arousal are monitored by electroencephalography, electrooculography, and electromyography. The NPSG is overseen by a skilled technician and interpreted by a sleep specialist. During the test, several physiologic markers are constantly monitored, including respiratory rate, air flow, oxygen saturation, chest wall movements, heart rate and rhythm, eye and limb movements, and brain activities. Data collected during the test are used to determine the AHI.

Ordinarily, patients with HF will have a predominant type of SDB, either obstructive or central. However, it is not uncommon to see both types coexist in the same patient. In the mixed type of SDB, a gradual shift from a dominate OSA at the beginning of the night to predominant CSA later in the night is often noticed.[5,72] This observation is attributed to worsening cardiac output as the night progresses.[5,72]

Although NPSG remains the gold standard and the most comprehensive method for testing patients with SDB, it has many challenges that limit its applicability. NPGS is expensive and time consuming and requires an overnight stay at a specialized laboratory, which can be inconvenient for many patients. As a result, there has been growing interest in alternative diagnostic tools such as portable sleep monitors.

Ambulatory sleep testing Several portable monitors have been proposed in recent years for the purpose of unattended home-based use. Those devices differ in the number of sleep markers they measure. The most widely used currently are the ambulatory cardiorespiratory testing devices.[73] Studies of class III devices, which measure nasal flow, oxygen saturation, and thoracic and abdominal movement have established an acceptable accuracy in diagnosing SDB and determining the type (OSA vs OSA) when compared with standard NPSG.[11,74]

Those devices are approved by Medicare for the diagnosis of OSA, and their results can justify the prescription of continuous positive airway pressure (CPAP). The concept of abbreviated sleep testing is increasingly gaining acceptance and will likely become the standard in patients with high pretest probability such as HF patients.[3,9,11] Major limitations of the portable devices are their inability to measure sleep, which could lead to underestimating SDB severity. Overnight pulse oximetry was once proposed as a screening tool for DSB, but this method was deemed inadequate in establishing the diagnosis because both OSA and CSA are not always associated with pronounced arterial oxygen desaturation.[75]

TREATMENT OF SLEEP-DISORDERED BREATHING IN HEART FAILURE PATIENTS

The treatment approach for SDB should follow a systematic, multidimensional strategy to ensure appropriate delivery of therapy and guarantee good compliance and long-term efficacy. In patients with HF, special attention should be paid to optimizing HF therapy. This is a key step in SDB management because of the reciprocal interactions between HF and OSA. Providers and patients should bear in mind that SDB treatment is not a one-time occurrence but rather a long-term commitment because of the chronicity of the disease. Additionally, the type of therapy should be guided by the result of sleep study and target the sleep disturbances mainly seen on PSG. Lastly, because the success of treatment highly depends on a high adherence rate, patients should be kept well informed about their therapeutic choices and viewed as an essential part in decision making.

Because practice guidelines lack integrated schemes to SDB management, we propose simplified practical approaches to aid practitioners in the treatment of the OSA and CSA, which are discussed below (**Figs. 1** and **2**).

TREATMENT OF OBSTRUCTIVE SLEEP APNEA

The first approach to HF patients with OSA should focus on optimization of HF medical therapy. Pulmonary and systemic congestions are the main manifestations of HF and major triggers of OSA exacerbation,[68,69] thus diuretics should be used aggressively to restore euvolemia. Guideline-directed medical therapy (GDMT) for HF should be instigated based on HF stage and functional class according to published guidelines and titrated to achieve the best therapeutic effects. GDMT includes treatment with BBs, which oppose the effects of sympathetic stimulation and treatment with angiotensin-converting enzyme inhibitors (ACEi) or angiotensin receptor blockers

(ARB), which oppose the effect of renin angiotensin system, augment vasodilation, and enhance cardiac performance. Aldosterone antagonists such as spironolactone or eplerenone are proven to improve morbidity and mortality in moderate-to-severe HF. Treatment with spironolactone is known to improve AHI in OSA by its effect on treating hypertension, restoring euvolemia, and improving postural fluid[76] and should be complementary to BB, ACEi, and ARB in the treatment of HF and OSA.[77]

Therapeutic options for OSA should be tailored in accordance to the severity of OSA-related sleep disturbances assessed by PSG. Mild cases can be adequately managed by behavioral changes and lifestyle modifications. These include weight loss among obese patients, avoidance of central nervous system suppressants, such as sedatives or alcoholic beverages, and encouraging comfortable sleep positions that prevent cranial and central fluid shift.[78] Among patients with moderate-to-severe OSA and those with mild OSA on PSG but symptomatic with presence of daytime sleepiness, treatment with CPAP is recommended.[78]

CPAP is a pneumatic device designed to provide positive pressure to the upper airway and proven to be highly effective in reducing obstruction and restoring patency. The device consists of electric air blower connected to tubing through which pressurized air is delivered to the patient through nasal or facial mask. CPAP therapeutic benefits in HF are believed to be mediated by improving oxygenation, blunting CNS stimulation, and normalization of intrathoracic pressures.[79–82]

In symptomatic patients with OSA, treatment with CPAP is effective in restoring normal sleep habits, reducing daytime sleepiness, and improving cognitive function.[83,84] Among HF patients with OSA, CPAP therapy was effective in reducing hypoxic events, normalizing nocturnal high blood pressure and tachycardia, and improving left ventricular function.[79–82] A small study suggested that treatment with CPAP could improve mortality and HF hospitalizations in HF patients with OSA,[85] but these findings were not validated in a large randomized trial that was published recently.[86] The SAVE trail was an international, multicenter, open-label trial with a blinded endpoint that randomly assigned 2717 patients between 45 and 75 year of age with moderate to severe OSA and other cardiovascular risk markers including history of coronary or cerebrovascular disease to receive treatment with CPAP or usual care.[86] After a mean follow-up of 3.7 years, there was no difference in primary composite endpoint of death from cardiovascular causes, myocardial infarction, stroke, or hospitalization for unstable

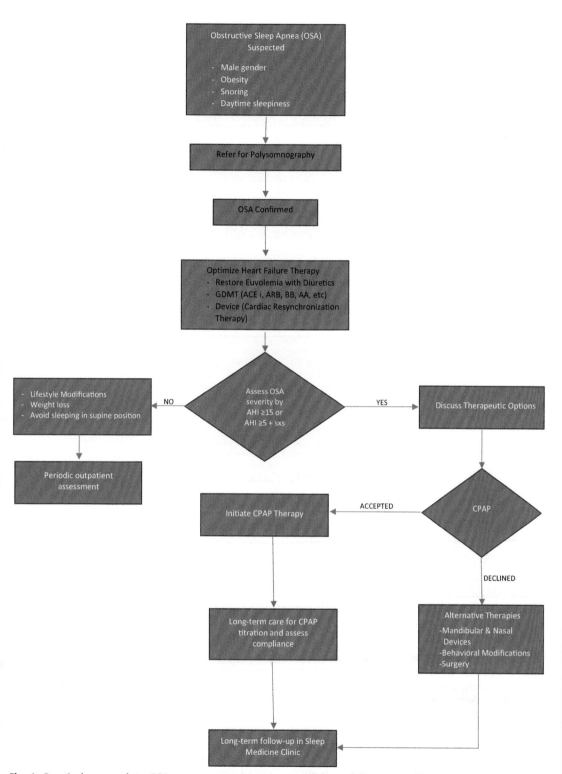

Fig. 1. Practical approach to OSA management in patients with heart failure. AA, aldosterone antagonists.

angina, HF, or transient ischemic attack. Average AHI was reduced in the CPAP arm from 29 events per hour to 3.9 events per hour. CPAP effectively reduced snoring and daytime sleepiness and improved health-related quality of life and mood. The SAVE trial has several limitations that could have influenced its result. First, the study was not powered to provide definitive conclusion

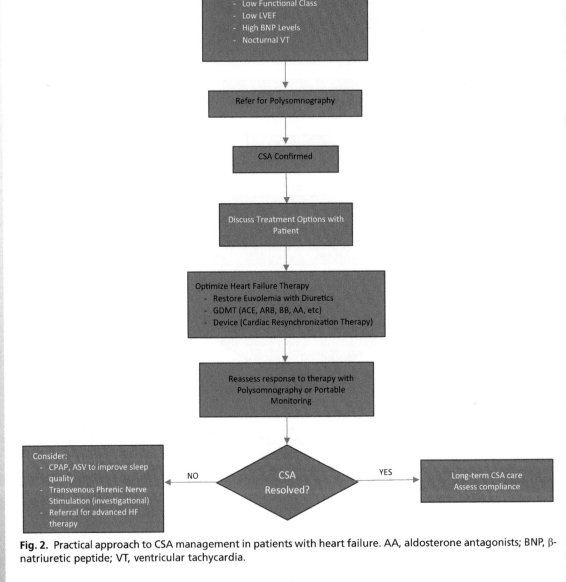

Fig. 2. Practical approach to CSA management in patients with heart failure. AA, aldosterone antagonists; BNP, β-natriuretic peptide; VT, ventricular tachycardia.

regarding CPAP effects on secondary cardiovascular endpoints. Second, there were significant practice variations among centers participating in the study; this was more pronounced in some participating countries in which the diagnosis and treatment of OSA was not well established when this trial was first started. Third, the average adherence to CPAP in the study is 3.3 hours per night, which is in line with prior CPAP trials in which patients had mild or no daytime sleepiness, but this duration could still be insufficient to influence cardiovascular outcomes.

Therapeutic benefits of CPAP depend highly on the duration of its use; thus, proper adherence to

therapy to meet the prescribed number of hours is perhaps the most important factor in therapeutic success. Poor compliance with CPAP therapy is a common problem; it tends to occur early and may affect half of the patients.[87] Causes for noncompliance include mask-related discomfort, nasal dryness, claustrophobia, anxiety, and panic attacks. These caused can be mitigated by mask adjustment and using humidification. Frequent follow-up and re-assessment of compliance are needed to ensure delivery of adequate therapy.

Besides CPAP, other alternative therapies for OSA have been proposed, including surgical procedures intended to enlarge the constricted upper airways and the application of mandibular and nasal devices designed to prevent tongue-mediated pharyngeal obstruction and widen the nostrils, respectively. Despite early enthusiasm, none of these therapies were found to be effective in the treatment of OSA,[78] and their use should be cautiously reserved to special cases when anatomic abnormality is the dominant etiology or when CPAP is ineffective or cannot be tolerated.

TREATMENT OF CENTRAL SLEEP APNEA

In general, treatment of CSA in HF has been less successful than OSA, and, as of today, there is no agreement on any effective therapeutic strategy for CSA. Several therapies have been proposed and studied in the CSA and HF populations. Early clinical trials found possible benefits in reducing CSA events and symptoms; however, none of these therapies was proven to be curative or associated with improved cardiovascular outcome.

CSA treatment should focus on addressing CSA itself and improving HF symptoms. Adequate management of HF is by far the most significant factor in controlling CSA, and numbers of clinical trials have shown parallel improvement in CSA once HF is improved.[88–91] In addition to medical therapy, treatment of HF should also encompass device-based therapy such as cardiac resynchronization therapy (CRT) in select patients. CRT, mediated by improvement in cardiac efficiency and cardiac output, was proven to reduce CSA events in eligible HF patients who received CRT devices.[91,92]

Most patients will continue to have residual CSA even after HF therapy is optimized, which can be addressed by CSA targeted therapy. CPAP was extensively studied in the CSA population, and data on its efficacy have not been established. Small early trials found possible benefits in reducing ventricular irritability, lessening SNA activity, improving quality of life, and possibly improving survival.[56,93–95] To confirm these findings in a large, prospective multicenter fashion, The Canadian Continuous Positive Airway Pressure for Central Sleep Apnea (CANPAP) and Heart Failure study was conducted.[96] This study was the largest study that tested whether treatment of CSA in the HF population would reduce mortality and improve transplant-free survival. After mean follow-up of 2 years, there was no difference in mortality, number of hospitalizations, quality of life, and brain natriuretic peptide levels. On the positive side, the AHI was reduced from 40 to 19 events per hour after 3 months of CPAP therapy, and this was associated with improved nighttime

oxygenation, exercise tolerance, and left ventricular ejection fraction.

One of the major limitations of the CANPAP trial was adherence to therapy. Compliance with CPAP was only 3.6 hours after 1 year of follow-up. In fact, post-hoc analysis of patients who achieved reduction of AHI to less than 15 events per hour showed statistically significant improvement in transplant-free survival.[97] Overall, CANPAP is regarded as a negative study, and based on its findings, the use of CPAP in patients with HF and CSA is not expected to improve survival.

Because of the inconsistent therapeutic effects of CPAP on CSA, a newer way of noninvasive ventilation called *adaptive-pressure support servoventilaiton* (ASV) was proposed. ASV functions similarly to CPAP and can deliver continuous positive pressure support, but it is also equipped with a sensor that detects central apnea events, during which it delivers several breaths at a rate and tidal volume calculated based on average in patients in stable condition. It was proposed that this extra feature would prevent the increase in $Paco_2$ during apneic events and lessen ventilatory overshoot phenomenon, thus breaking the self-perpetuated periodic breathing cycles.

ASV use on average gains better acceptance by most patients.[98–100] This is perhaps because of ASV dynamic control of pressure support based on the nature of sleep disturbances detected by the AVS sensor, which enhance the regulation of airflow. Small clinical trials found superior effect of ASV over CPAP in reducing CSA in HF with improvement in cardiac function and quality of life.[98–100] However, this earlier excitement with regard to ASV improved outcome received a major drawback after the release of a large multinational trial that evaluated AVS effects on morbidity and mortality in patients with reduced ejection fraction and CSA.[101] This study, called SERVE-HF,[101] did not find survival benefit from treatment of CSA in HF patients. It rather showed increased mortality in the treatment by an exploratory analysis that was not controlled for type I error. To explain that, it was proposed that CSA could represent a compensatory mechanism in HF and any attempt to correct it by ASV, or possibly any other means, would incite harmful consequences.

The concept of CSA as a compensatory mechanism in heart failure with reduced ejection fraction (HFrEF) was based on the observation that CSR is associated with hyperventilation-related increases in end-expiratory lung volume, intrinsic positive airway pressure, and possible decrease of work of breathing.[102] This notion was never tested directly in humans with HF, however. Furthermore, it stands in opposition to numerous studies over the last few decades showing a negative impact of CSA in HFrEF patients. Although, the treatment of CSA with CPAP and ASV has not been shown to improve mortality in HF patients, the neuro-humoral consequences of CSA and their elimination with treatment are well documented in HF patients.[56,62,103,104] Notably, several of the hypothesized compensatory mechanisms of CSA would also be achieved by the application of positive airway pressure: CPAP or ASV, which should have led to strongly positive outcomes in randomized trials using these modalities. Furthermore, central events are associated with airway collapse at the end of apnea,[105] and the clinical definition of CSA can include patients with a substantial number of obstructive events.[106,107] Also, both OSA and CSA are associated with a cyclical breathing pattern with variations in the amount of obstruction from night to night. Therefore, a decision not to treat a patient with HF and CSA is not justified and would leave this patient exposed to unmitigated hypoxia, sympathetic activation, disturbed sleep, and arrhythmia.

Therefore, the current trial findings support that treatment of CSA with ASV in patients with low ejection fraction is not beneficial and is possibly harmful. The available trials do not support that CPAP is associated with harm in this population, however. The mechanism by which ASV may be associated with harm in patients with HF and reduced EF is discussed elsewhere in this special issue and was addressed in publications recently.[108,109]

Modalities other than positive airway pressure for the treatment of CSA are discussed in a dedicated article in this special issue but few emerging treatment options are important for us to briefly note.

Unilateral stimulation of the phrenic nerve via pacing devices is an innovative therapy for CSA. The system is fully implanted and used pulse generator and 2 pacing leads, one for sensing and the other for stimulation. The principle of this therapy is based on the fact that stimulation of the phrenic nerve during an apneic episode will provide adequate ventilation; therefore, it will prevent hypocapnea and the subsequent ventilatory overshoot.[110] Data with this modality have been encouraging with benefits seen in decreasing CSA events and arousals, improving oxygenation and quality of life.[111]

Several pharmacologic therapies have been proposed in the treatment of CSA. Those agents share the same stimulatory effects on the central ventilatory system. It was proposed that by their ability to increase ventilation and CO_2 reserve, they can decrease the ventilatory overshoot and diminish the possibility of apnea after arousals.

Theophylline is a known respiratory stimulant and one of the early drugs used in the treatment of CSA in HF. In a small study with short follow-up, theophylline was found to decrease central apnea and oxyhemoglobin desaturation with no change noted in the left ventricular ejection fraction (LVEF) when it was compared with placebo in HF patients with CSA.[112] Theophylline, however, has a very narrow therapeutic window and its use causes tachycardia. Thus, its use in HF should be taken with extreme caution.

Acetazolamide is a weak diuretic that was proposed in the treatment of CSA because of its ability to cause metabolic acidosis. The body compensates for the metabolic acidosis by decreasing $Paco_2$. This will subsequently increase the margin above which $Paco_2$ reaches the apneic threshold, which leads to decreasing the likelihood of CSA development.[113]

In a small, double-blind, prospective trial with short follow-up that enrolled HF patients with CSA, acetazolamide decreased respiratory events, reduced the severity of nocturnal oxygen desaturation, and improved subjective markers of sleep quality when compared with placebo. In this trial, acetazolamide use was not associated with improved objective measures of sleep quality and LVEF.[114] Acetazolamide provokes urinary potassium wasting leading to hypokalemia, which can increase arrhythmia risk, and its use is generally discouraged in HF patients.

Benzodiazepines and other hypnotics were considered in the treatment of CSA with proposed mechanism of blunting ventilatory overshoot. Small studies found a decrease in the number of nocturnal arousals, but there was no effect in the severity of respiratory events or nocturnal oxyhemoglobin desaturation.[115,116]

The stimulatory effect of carbon dioxide on the ventilatory control system has been evaluated as therapeutic potential in CSA treatment. Carbon dioxide can lessen periodic breathing cycles by increasing baseline ventilation and the margin between baseline $Paco_2$ and apnea threshold. The increased ventilatory drive can further enhance upper airway patency.[117,118] Data on long term efficacy of carbon dioxide in the treatment of CSA in HF are lacking, and safety of its use and delivery is of major concern.[119]

SUMMARY

It is estimated that more than two-thirds of patients with HF have SDB. Although OSA coexists with all stages of HF and shares many predisposing risk factors, CSA is considered a marker of advanced HF state and more prevalent in severe cases. Both types of SDB produce a cyclical pattern of apnea and hypopnea episodes that have detrimental vascular and hemodynamic effects on the cardiovascular system mediated by changes in intrathoracic pressures, activation of the sympathetic nervous system, and creation of an intensified inflammatory milieu. HF patients with SDB have a worse prognosis compared with those without SDB. High index of suspicion for SDB should be always implemented on approaching patients with HF because of similarity of SDB symptoms and other HF symptoms including medication side effect. Patient screening should be followed by a sleep study to confirm the diagnosis and assess the severity of the disease. Mild cases of OSA can be managed by lifestyle modifications and restoring euvolemic state. Severe cases of OSA should be offered CPAP therapy, which is proven to improve symptoms and cardiac function and attenuate sympathetic activities. CPAP therapy, however, was not associated with reduction in HF mortality and morbidity when tested in a randomized fashion. This finding could be influenced by duration of CPAP therapy and practice variations. More data are needed to clarify the roles of CPAP therapy in HF patients. Similarly, positive pressure devices (CPAP and ASV) were tested in the treatment of CSA in HF in a randomized fashion and yielded no benefits. In fact, there was trend toward increased mortality with ASV use, which was attributed to the negative effect of positive pressure support on cardiopulmonary hemodynamics. Duration of use effect for ASV devices could have influenced the outcome and should be further evaluated. As of today, with the lack of effective therapy, CSA should be considered a consequence of advanced HF and is best treated with greater focus on optimizing HF medical and device-based therapies. Phrenic nerve stimulation is an intriguing approach for CSA and may offer a therapeutic breakthrough. Their full efficacy is yet to be determined.

REFERENCES

1. Javaheri S, Parker TJ, Liming JD, et al. Sleep apnea in 81 ambulatory male patients with stable heart failure. Types and their prevalences, consequences, and presentations. Circulation 1998; 97(21):2154–9.
2. Paulino A, Damy T, Margarit L, et al. Prevalence of sleep-disordered breathing in a 316-patient French cohort of stable congestive heart failure. Arch Cardiovasc Dis 2009;102(3):169–75.
3. Oldenburg O, Lamp B, Faber L, et al. Sleep-disordered breathing in patients with symptomatic heart failure: a contemporary study of prevalence in and characteristics of 700 patients. Eur J Heart Fail 2007;9(3):251–7.
4. Javaheri S, Caref EB, Chen E, et al. Sleep apnea testing and outcomes in a large cohort of Medicare beneficiaries with newly diagnosed heart failure. Am J Respir Crit Care Med 2011;183(4):539–46.
5. Tkacova R, Wang H, Bradley TD. Night-to-night alterations in sleep apnea type in patients with heart failure. J Sleep Res 2006;15(3):321–8.
6. Young T, Palta M, Dempsey J, et al. The occurrence of sleep-disordered breathing among middle-aged adults. N Engl J Med 1993;328(17):1230–5.
7. Ancoli-Israel S, Kripke DF, Klauber MR, et al. Sleep-disordered breathing in community-dwelling elderly. Sleep 1991;14(6):486–95.
8. Lorenzi-Filho G, Dajani HR, Leung RS, et al. Entrainment of blood pressure and heart rate oscillations by periodic breathing. Am J Respir Crit Care Med 1999;159(4 Pt 1):1147–54.
9. Schulz R, Blau A, Borgel J, et al. Sleep apnoea in heart failure. Eur Respir J 2007;29(6):1201–5.
10. Tamura A, Kawano Y, Naono S, et al. Relationship between beta-blocker treatment and the severity of central sleep apnea in chronic heart failure. Chest 2007;131(1):130–5.
11. Khayat RN, Jarjoura D, Patt B, et al. In-hospital testing for sleep-disordered breathing in hospitalized patients with decompensated heart failure: report of prevalence and patient characteristics. J Card Fail 2009;15(9):739–46.
12. Marin JM, Carrizo SJ, Vicente E, et al. Long-term cardiovascular outcomes in men with obstructive sleep apnoea-hypopnoea with or without treatment with continuous positive airway pressure: an observational study. Lancet 2005;365(9464):1046–53.
13. Young T, Peppard P, Palta M, et al. Population-based study of sleep-disordered breathing as a risk factor for hypertension. Arch Intern Med 1997;157(15):1746–52.
14. Millman RP, Redline S, Carlisle CC, et al. Daytime hypertension in obstructive sleep apnea. Prevalence and contributing risk factors. Chest 1991; 99(4):861–6.
15. Chan J, Sanderson J, Chan W, et al. Prevalence of sleep-disordered breathing in diastolic heart failure. Chest 1997;111(6):1488–93.
16. Zhou XS, Rowley JA, Demirovic F, et al. Effect of testosterone on the apneic threshold in women during NREM sleep. J Appl Physiol 2003;94(1): 101–7.
17. Tishler PV, Larkin EK, Schluchter MD, et al. Incidence of sleep-disordered breathing in an urban adult population: the relative importance of risk factors in the development of sleep-disordered breathing. JAMA 2003;289(17):2230–7.
18. Morgan BJ, Denahan T, Ebert TJ. Neurocirculatory consequences of negative intrathoracic pressure

vs. asphyxia during voluntary apnea. J Appl Physiol 1993;74(6):2969–75.

19. Katragadda S, Xie A, Puleo D, et al. Neural mechanism of the pressor response to obstructive and nonobstructive apnea. J Appl Physiol 1997;83(6):2048–54.

20. Peng YJ, Prabhakar NR. Reactive oxygen species in the plasticity of respiratory behavior elicited by chronic intermittent hypoxia. J Appl Physiol 2003; 94(6):2342–9.

21. Prabhakar NR, Fields RD, Baker T, et al. Intermittent hypoxia: cell to system. Am J Physiol Lung Cell Mol Physiol 2001;281(3):L524–8.

22. Prabhakar NR, Kline DD. Ventilatory changes during intermittent hypoxia: importance of pattern and duration. High Alt Med Biol 2002; 3(2):195–204.

23. Cutler MJ, Swift NM, Keller DM, et al. Periods of intermittent hypoxic apnea can alter chemoreflex control of sympathetic nerve activity in humans. Am J Physiol Heart Circ Physiol 2004;287(5): H2054–60.

24. Lesske J, Fletcher EC, Bao G, et al. Hypertension caused by chronic intermittent hypoxia–influence of chemoreceptors and sympathetic nervous system. J Hypertens 1997;15(12 Pt 2):1593–603.

25. Fletcher EC. Invited review: physiological consequences of intermittent hypoxia: systemic blood pressure. J Appl Physiol 2001;90(4):1600–5.

26. Brooks D, Horner RL, Kozar LF, et al. Obstructive sleep apnea as a cause of systemic hypertension. Evidence from a canine model. J Clin Invest 1997; 99(1):106–9.

27. Peppard PE, Young T, Palta M, et al. Prospective study of the association between sleep-disordered breathing and hypertension. N Engl J Med 2000;342(19):1378–84.

28. Leung RS, Bradley TD. Sleep apnea and cardiovascular disease. Am J Respir Crit Care Med 2001;164(12):2147–65.

29. Hung J, Whitford EG, Parsons RW, et al. Association of sleep apnoea with myocardial infarction in men. Lancet 1990;336(8710):261–4.

30. Yumino D, Tsurumi Y, Takagi A, et al. Impact of obstructive sleep apnea on clinical and angiographic outcomes following percutaneous coronary intervention in patients with acute coronary syndrome. Am J Cardiol 2007;99(1):26–30.

31. Peker Y, Hedner J, Kraiczi H, et al. Respiratory disturbance index: an independent predictor of mortality in coronary artery disease. Am J Respir Crit Care Med 2000;162(1):81–6.

32. Gami AS, Pressman G, Caples SM, et al. Association of atrial fibrillation and obstructive sleep apnea. Circulation 2004;110(4):364–7.

33. Kanagala R, Murali NS, Friedman PA, et al. Obstructive sleep apnea and the recurrence of atrial fibrillation. Circulation 2003;107(20):2589–94.

34. Shahar E, Whitney CW, Redline S, et al. Sleep-disordered breathing and cardiovascular disease: cross-sectional results of the Sleep Heart Health Study. Am J Respir Crit Care Med 2001;163(1): 19–25.

35. Bradley TD, Hall MJ, Ando S, et al. Hemodynamic effects of simulated obstructive apneas in humans with and without heart failure. Chest 2001;119(6): 1827–35.

36. Brinker JA, Weiss JL, Lappe DL, et al. Leftward septal displacement during right ventricular loading in man. Circulation 1980;61(3):626–33.

37. Franklin KA, Nilsson JB, Sahlin C, et al. Sleep apnoea and nocturnal angina. Lancet 1995; 345(8957):1085–7.

38. Larkin EK, Rosen CL, Kirchner HL, et al. Variation of C-reactive protein levels in adolescents: association with sleep-disordered breathing and sleep duration. Circulation 2005;111(15):1978–84.

39. Gottlieb DJ, Yenokyan G, Newman AB, et al. Prospective study of obstructive sleep apnea and incident coronary heart disease and heart failure: the sleep heart health study. Circulation 2010;122(4): 352–60.

40. Javaheri S. Sleep disorders in systolic heart failure: a prospective study of 100 male patients. The final report. Int J Cardiol 2006;106(1):21–8.

41. Sin DD, Fitzgerald F, Parker JD, et al. Risk factors for central and obstructive sleep apnea in 450 men and women with congestive heart failure. Am J Respir Crit Care Med 1999;160(4):1101–6.

42. MacDonald M, Fang J, Pittman SD, et al. The current prevalence of sleep disordered breathing in congestive heart failure patients treated with beta-blockers. J Clin Sleep Med 2008;4(1):38–42.

43. Herrscher TE, Akre H, Overland B, et al. High prevalence of sleep apnea in heart failure outpatients: even in patients with preserved systolic function. J Card Fail 2011;17(5):420–5.

44. Bitter T, Langer C, Vogt J, et al. Sleep-disordered breathing in patients with atrial fibrillation and normal systolic left ventricular function. Dtsch Arztebl Int 2009;106(10):164–70.

45. Naughton M, Benard D, Tam A, et al. Role of hyperventilation in the pathogenesis of central sleep apneas in patients with congestive heart failure. Am Rev Respir Dis 1993;148(2):330–8.

46. Hanly P, Zuberi N, Gray R. Pathogenesis of Cheyne-Stokes respiration in patients with congestive heart failure. Relationship to arterial PCO2. Chest 1993;104(4):1079–84.

47. Dempsey JA. Crossing the apnoeic threshold: causes and consequences. Exp Physiol 2005; 90(1):13–24.

48. Naughton MT, Bradley TD. Sleep apnea in congestive heart failure. Clin Chest Med 1998; 19(1):99–113.

49. Xie A, Skatrud JB, Khayat R, et al. Cerebrovascular response to carbon dioxide in patients with congestive heart failure. Am J Respir Crit Care Med 2005;172(3):371–8.

50. Alex CG, Onal E, Lopata M. Upper airway occlusion during sleep in patients with Cheyne-Stokes respiration. Am Rev Respir Dis 1986;133(1):42–5.

51. Badr MS, Toiber F, Skatrud JB, et al. Pharyngeal narrowing/occlusion during central sleep apnea. J Appl Physiol (1985) 1995;78(5):1806–15.

52. Hall MJ, Xie A, Rutherford R, et al. Cycle length of periodic breathing in patients with and without heart failure. Am J Respir Crit Care Med 1996; 154(2 Pt 1):376–81.

53. Somers VK, Mark AL, Zavala DC, et al. Contrasting effects of hypoxia and hypercapnia on ventilation and sympathetic activity in humans. J Appl Physiol (1985) 1989;67(5):2101–6.

54. Kaye DM, Lefkovits J, Jennings GL, et al. Adverse consequences of high sympathetic nervous activity in the failing human heart. J Am Coll Cardiol 1995; 26(5):1257–63.

55. Leung RS, Diep TM, Bowman ME, et al. Provocation of ventricular ectopy by cheyne-stokes respiration in patients with heart failure. Sleep 2004;27(7): 1337–43.

56. Sin DD, Logan AG, Fitzgerald FS, et al. Effects of continuous positive airway pressure on cardiovascular outcomes in heart failure patients with and without Cheyne-Stokes respiration. Circulation 2000;102(1):61–6.

57. Trinder J, Merson R, Rosenberg JI, et al. Pathophysiological interactions of ventilation, arousals, and blood pressure oscillations during cheyne-stokes respiration in patients with heart failure. Am J Respir Crit Care Med 2000;162(3 Pt 1): 808–13.

58. Lanfranchi PA, Somers VK, Braghiroli A, et al. Central sleep apnea in left ventricular dysfunction: prevalence and implications for arrhythmic risk. Circulation 2003;107(5):727–32.

59. Hanly PJ, Zuberi-Khokhar NS. Increased mortality associated with Cheyne-Stokes respiration in patients with congestive heart failure. Am J Respir Crit Care Med 1996;153(1):272–6.

60. Lanfranchi PA, Braghiroli A, Bosimini E, et al. Prognostic value of nocturnal Cheyne-Stokes respiration in chronic heart failure. Circulation 1999; 99(11):1435–40.

61. Khayat R, Abraham W, Patt B, et al. Central sleep apnea is a predictor of cardiac readmission in hospitalized patients with systolic heart failure. J Card Fail 2012;18(7):534–40.

62. Naughton MT, Benard DC, Liu PP, et al. Effects of nasal CPAP on sympathetic activity in patients with heart failure and central sleep apnea. Am J Respir Crit Care Med 1995;152(2):473–9.

63. Johns MW. A new method for measuring daytime sleepiness: the Epworth sleepiness scale. Sleep 1991;14(6):540–5.

64. Johns MW. Sleepiness in different situations measured by the Epworth sleepiness scale. Sleep 1994;17(8):703–10.

65. Netzer NC, Stoohs RA, Netzer CM, et al. Using the Berlin Questionnaire to identify patients at risk for the sleep apnea syndrome. Ann Intern Med 1999; 131(7):485–91.

66. Arzt M, Young T, Finn L, et al. Sleepiness and sleep in patients with both systolic heart failure and obstructive sleep apnea. Arch Intern Med 2006; 166(16):1716–22.

67. Schwab RJ, Pasirstein M, Pierson R, et al. Identification of upper airway anatomic risk factors for obstructive sleep apnea with volumetric magnetic resonance imaging. Am J Respir Crit Care Med 2003;168(5):522–30.

68. Friedman O, Bradley TD, Chan CT, et al. Relationship between overnight rostral fluid shift and obstructive sleep apnea in drug-resistant hypertension. Hypertension 2010;56(6):1077–82.

69. Redolfi S, Yumino D, Ruttanaumpawan P, et al. Relationship between overnight rostral fluid shift and Obstructive Sleep Apnea in nonobese men. Am J Respir Crit Care Med 2009;179(3):241–6.

70. Nuckton TJ, Glidden DV, Browner WS, et al. Physical examination: Mallampati score as an independent predictor of obstructive sleep apnea. Sleep 2006;29(7):903–8.

71. Oldenburg O, Lamp B, Topfer V, et al. Prevalence of sleep-related breathing disorders in ischemic and non-ischemic heart failure. Dtsch Med Wochenschr 2007;132(13):661–6.

72. Tkacova R, Niroumand M, Lorenzi-Filho G, et al. Overnight shift from obstructive to central apneas in patients with heart failure: role of PCO2 and circulatory delay. Circulation 2001;103(2): 238–43.

73. Nancy A, Collop WMA, Boehlecke B, et al. Portable monitoring task force for the American Academy of Sleep Medicine. Clinical guidelines for the use of unattended portable monitors in the diagnosis of obstructive sleep apnea in adult patients. J Clin Sleep Med 2007;3(7):737–47.

74. Quintana-Gallego E, Villa-Gil M, Carmona-Bernal C, et al. Home respiratory polygraphy for diagnosis of sleep-disordered breathing in heart failure. Eur Respir J 2004;24(3):443–8.

75. Flemons WW, Littner MR, Rowley JA, et al. Home diagnosis of sleep apnea: a systematic review of the literature. An evidence review cosponsored by the American Academy of Sleep Medicine, the American College of Chest Physicians, and the American Thoracic Society. Chest 2003;124(4): 1543–79.

76. Gaddam K, Pimenta E, Thomas SJ, et al. Spirono-lactone reduces severity of obstructive sleep apnoea in patients with resistant hypertension: a preliminary report. J Hum Hypertens 2010;24(8): 532–7.

77. Hunt SA, Abraham WT, Chin MH, et al. 2009 focused update incorporated into the ACC/AHA 2005 guidelines for the diagnosis and management of heart failure in adults a report of the American College of Cardiology Foundation/American Heart Association Task Force on Practice Guidelines Developed in Collaboration With the International Society for Heart and Lung Transplantation. J Am Coll Cardiol 2009;53(15):e1–90.

78. Epstein LJ, Kristo D, Strollo PJ Jr, et al. Clinical guideline for the evaluation, management and long-term care of obstructive sleep apnea in adults. J Clin Sleep Med 2009;5(3):263–76.

79. Tkacova R, Rankin F, Fitzgerald FS, et al. Effects of continuous positive airway pressure on obstructive sleep apnea and left ventricular afterload in patients with heart failure. Circulation 1998;98(21):2269–75.

80. Malone S, Liu PP, Holloway R, et al. Obstructive sleep apnoea in patients with dilated cardiomyopathy: effects of continuous positive airway pressure. Lancet 1991;338(8781):1480–4.

81. Kaneko Y, Floras JS, Usui K, et al. Cardiovascular effects of continuous positive airway pressure in patients with heart failure and obstructive sleep apnea. N Engl J Med 2003;348(13):1233–41.

82. Mansfield DR, Gollogly NC, Kaye DM, et al. Controlled trial of continuous positive airway pressure in obstructive sleep apnea and heart failure. Am J Respir Crit Care Med 2004;169(3):361–6.

83. Engleman HM, Martin SE, Deary IJ, et al. Effect of continuous positive airway pressure treatment on daytime function in sleep apnoea/hypopnoea syndrome. Lancet 1994;343(8897):572–5.

84. Engleman HM, Kingshott RN, Wraith PK, et al. Randomized placebo-controlled crossover trial of continuous positive airway pressure for mild sleep Apnea/Hypopnea syndrome. Am J Respir Crit Care Med 1999;159(2):461–7.

85. Kasai T, Narui K, Dohi T, et al. Prognosis of patients with heart failure and obstructive sleep apnea treated with continuous positive airway pressure. Chest 2008;133(3):690–6.

86. McEvoy RD, Antic NA, Heeley E, et al. CPAP for prevention of cardiovascular events in obstructive sleep apnea. N Engl J Med 2016;375(10):919–31.

87. Indications and standards for use of nasal continuous positive airway pressure (CPAP) in sleep apnea syndromes. American Thoracic Society. Official statement adopted March 1944. Am J Respir Crit Care Med 1994;150(6 Pt 1):1738–45.

88. Dark DS, Pingleton SK, Kerby GR, et al. Breathing pattern abnormalities and arterial oxygen desaturation during sleep in the congestive heart failure syndrome. Improvement following medical therapy. Chest 1987;91(6):833–6.

89. Walsh JT, Andrews R, Starling R, et al. Effects of captopril and oxygen on sleep apnoea in patients with mild to moderate congestive cardiac failure. Br Heart J 1995;73(3):237–41.

90. Baylor P, Tayloe D, Owen D, et al. Cardiac failure presenting as sleep apnea. Elimination of apnea following medical management of cardiac failure. Chest 1988;94(6):1298–300.

91. Sinha AM, Skobel EC, Breithardt OA, et al. Cardiac resynchronization therapy improves central sleep apnea and Cheyne-Stokes respiration in patients with chronic heart failure. J Am Coll Cardiol 2004; 44(1):68–71.

92. Kara T, Novak M, Nykodym J, et al. Short-term effects of cardiac resynchronization therapy on sleep-disordered breathing in patients with systolic heart failure. Chest 2008;134(1):87–93.

93. Javaheri S. Effects of continuous positive airway pressure on sleep apnea and ventricular irritability in patients with heart failure. Circulation 2000; 101(4):392–7.

94. Naughton MT, Liu PP, Bernard DC, et al. Treatment of congestive heart failure and Cheyne-Stokes respiration during sleep by continuous positive airway pressure. Am J Respir Crit Care Med 1995;151(1):92–7.

95. Tkacova R, Liu PP, Naughton MT, et al. Effect of continuous positive airway pressure on mitral regurgitant fraction and atrial natriuretic peptide in patients with heart failure. J Am Coll Cardiol 1997;30(3):739–45.

96. Bradley TD, Logan AG, Kimoff RJ, et al. Continuous positive airway pressure for central sleep apnea and heart failure. N Engl J Med 2005;353(19): 2025–33.

97. Arzt M, Floras JS, Logan AG, et al. Suppression of central sleep apnea by continuous positive airway pressure and transplant-free survival in heart failure: a post hoc analysis of the Canadian Continuous Positive Airway Pressure for Patients with Central Sleep Apnea and Heart Failure Trial (CANPAP). Circulation 2007;115(25):3173–80.

98. Philippe C, Stoica-Herman M, Drouot X, et al. Compliance with and effectiveness of adaptive servoventilation versus continuous positive airway pressure in the treatment of Cheyne-Stokes respiration in heart failure over a six month period. Heart 2006;92(3):337–42.

99. Kasai T, Usui Y, Yoshioka T, et al. Effect of flow-triggered adaptive servo-ventilation compared with continuous positive airway pressure in patients with chronic heart failure with coexisting obstructive sleep apnea and Cheyne-Stokes respiration. Circ Heart Fail 2010;3(1):140–8.

100. Teschler H, Dohring J, Wang YM, et al. Adaptive pressure support servo-ventilation: a novel treatment for Cheyne-Stokes respiration in heart failure. Am J Respir Crit Care Med 2001;164(4):614–9.

101. Cowie MR, Woehrle H, Wegscheider K, et al. Adaptive servo-ventilation for central sleep apnea in systolic heart failure. N Engl J Med 2015;373(12):1095–105.

102. Naughton MT. Cheyne-Stokes respiration: friend or foe? Thorax 2012;67(4):357–60.

103. Kasai T, Narui K, Dohi T, et al. Efficacy of nasal bilevel positive airway pressure in congestive heart failure patients with cheyne-stokes respiration and central sleep apnea. Circ J 2005;69(8):913–21.

104. Granton JT, Naughton MT, Benard DC, et al. CPAP improves inspiratory muscle strength in patients with heart failure and central sleep apnea. Am J Respir Crit Care Med 1996;153(1):277–82.

105. Badr MS, Toiber F, Skatrud JB, et al. Pharyngeal narrowing/occlusion during central sleep apnea. J Appl Physiol 1995;78(5):1806–15.

106. Berry RB, Budhiraja R, Gottlieb DJ, et al. Rules for scoring respiratory events in sleep: update of the 2007 AASM manual for the scoring of sleep and associated events. Deliberations of the sleep apnea definitions task force of the American Academy of Sleep Medicine. J Clin Sleep Med 2012;8(5):597–619.

107. Ruehland WR, Rochford PD, O'Donoghue FJ, et al. The new AASM criteria for scoring hypopneas: impact on the apnea hypopnea index. Sleep 2009;32(2):150–7.

108. Javaheri S, Brown LK, Randerath W, et al. SERVE-HF: more questions than answers. Chest 2016;149(4):900–4.

109. Khayat RN, Abraham WT. Current treatment approaches and trials in central sleep apnea. Int J Cardiol 2016;206(Suppl):S22–7.

110. Costanzo MR, Ponikowski P, Javaheri S, et al. Transvenous neurostimulation for central sleep apnoea: a randomised controlled trial. Lancet 2016;388(10048):974–82.

111. Ponikowski P, Javaheri S, Michalkiewicz D, et al. Transvenous phrenic nerve stimulation for the treatment of central sleep apnoea in heart failure. Eur Heart J 2012;33(7):889–94.

112. Javaheri S, Parker TJ, Wexler L, et al. Effect of theophylline on sleep-disordered breathing in heart failure. N Engl J Med 1996;335(8):562–7.

113. White DP, Zwillich CW, Pickett CK, et al. Central sleep apnea. Improvement with acetazolamide therapy. Arch Intern Med 1982;142(10):1816–9.

114. Javaheri S. Acetazolamide improves central sleep apnea in heart failure: a double-blind, prospective study. Am J Respir Crit Care Med 2006;173(2):234–7.

115. Biberdorf DJ, Steens R, Millar TW, et al. Benzodiazepines in congestive heart failure: effects of temazepam on arousability and Cheyne-Stokes respiration. Sleep 1993;16(6):529–38.

116. Guilleminault C, Clerk A, Labanowski M, et al. Cardiac failure and benzodiazepines. Sleep 1993;16(6):524–8.

117. Dempsey JA, Veasey SC, Morgan BJ, et al. Pathophysiology of sleep apnea. Physiol Rev 2010;90(1):47–112.

118. Xie A, Teodorescu M, Pegelow DF, et al. Effects of stabilizing or increasing respiratory motor outputs on obstructive sleep apnea. J Appl Physiol (1985) 2013;115(1):22–33.

119. Khayat RN, Xie A, Patel AK, et al. Cardiorespiratory effects of added dead space in patients with heart failure and central sleep apnea. Chest 2003;123(5):1551–60.

Central Sleep Apnea in Patients with Congestive Heart Failure

James A. Rowley, MD[a],*, M. Safwan Badr, MD[b]

KEYWORDS

- Central sleep apnea • Congestive heart failure • Loop gain • Peripheral chemoreceptors
- Central chemoreceptors • Rostral fluid shifts

KEY POINTS

- Central sleep apnea (CSA) and Cheyne-Stokes respiration (CSR) are common in congestive heart failure (CHF).
- Common risk factors for CSA/CSR in patients with CHF are male gender, older age, hypocapnia, and the presence of atrial fibrillation.
- CSA arises from perturbations in the control of $Paco_2$ during the night.
- Augmented peripheral and central chemoreceptor activity is common in CHF and thought to underlie the perturbations in control of $Paco_2$ during sleep.
- Other important contributors to CSA/CSR in patients with CHF include rostral fluids shifts, diminished cerebrovascular activity, and prolonged circulation time.

Central sleep apnea (CSA) and Cheyne-Stokes respiration (CSR) during sleep are common in patients with congestive heart failure (CHF), representing a manifestation of breathing instability. This article reviews the determinants of CSA, the specific features of CHF-related CSA, and the underlying mechanisms.

DETERMINANTS OF BREATHING INSTABILITY DURING NON–RAPID EYE MOVEMENT SLEEP
Determinants of Central Apnea During Sleep

Breathing during wakefulness is influenced by both metabolic and behavioral factors. The sleep state (specifically non–rapid eye movement [NREM] sleep) is associated with loss of the wakefulness drive to breathe, rendering respiration critically dependent on chemical influences, especially $Paco_2$. Accordingly, a change in arterial $Paco_2$ leads to a corresponding change in ventilation to maintain the prevailing $Paco_2$ within a narrow physiologic range. However, CSA occurs if the arterial $Paco_2$ decreases below a reproducible sensitive hypocapnic apneic threshold.[1] Thus, hypocapnia is an important inhibitory factor during NREM sleep and is a key reason for the genesis of CSA and CSR in patients with CHF.[2]

CSA is common at sleep onset as the electroencephalogram oscillates between wakefulness and light sleep, with reciprocal changes in the $Paco_2$ around the apneic threshold. Thus, sleep state and breathing continue to oscillate until sleep is consolidated, a higher $Paco_2$ set point is established, and $Paco_2$ is maintained above this level.

Disclosure: The authors have nothing to disclose.

[a] Division of Pulmonary, Critical Care & Sleep Medicine, Harper University Hospital, Wayne State University School of Medicine, 3990 John R, 3 Hudson, Detroit, MI 48201, USA; [b] Division of Pulmonary, Critical Care & Sleep Medicine, Harper University Hospital, John D. Dingell VAMC, Wayne State University School of Medicine, 3990 John R, 3 Hudson, Detroit, MI 48201, USA
* Corresponding author.
E-mail address: jrowley@med.wayne.edu

Sleep Med Clin 12 (2017) 221–227
http://dx.doi.org/10.1016/j.jsmc.2017.03.001
1556-407X/17/© 2017 Elsevier Inc. All rights reserved.

CSA at sleep onset is described as physiologic; however, it is not universal. Thus, it is unclear whether CSA at sleep onset is a physiologic phenomenon or a subclinical marker of increased propensity to hypocapnic CSA.

CSA is uncommon during rapid eye movement (REM) sleep relative to NREM sleep. REM sleep may be impervious to central hypocapnic disfacilitation because central respiratory activity is increased during REM sleep,[3] suggesting that REM sleep is similar to wakefulness in terms of hypocapnic ventilatory response. Although post-hyperventilation CSA is rare in REM sleep, transient hypoventilation secondary to REM-induced loss of intercostal muscle activity in patients with neuromuscular disease may appear as CSA morphologically.

Determinants of Periodic Breathing During Sleep

CSA rarely occurs as a single event; instead, it occurs in cycles of apnea or hypopnea, alternating with hyperpnea, a reflection of the negative feedback closed-loop cycle that characterizes ventilatory control. Specifically, a transient change in chemical stimuli leads to a corresponding change in ventilation to correct the initial perturbation. Likewise, a transient increase in minute ventilation results in increased alveolar P_{O_2} and decreased P_{CO_2} and a subsequent ventilatory response, opposite to the initial perturbation. The overarching goal is to preserve ventilation and chemical stimuli within a narrow range, while responding to changes in sleep state or gas exchange, under a variety of physiologic or pathologic conditions. This process is often described using the engineering concept of loop gain, combining the response of the ventilatory system to changing partial pressure of end-tidal CO_2 ($P_{ET}CO_2$) (the controller), and the effectiveness of the lung/respiratory system in lowering $P_{ET}CO_2$ in response to hyperventilation (the plant).[4] Changes in either parameter change the requisite magnitude of hypocapnia to reach CSA (termed the CO_2 reserve; a lower CO_2 reserve is associated with an increased tendency to CSA). Loop gain is a useful concept in understanding control of breathing; however, the applicability of loop gain clinically is limited in part because arousals and upper airway obstruction can abruptly alter the responsiveness of the system to a perturbation in chemical stimuli.

Plant gain is the relationship between Δ P_{aCO_2} versus minute ventilation (Δ VE). It measures the efficacy of the system to change arterial P_{aCO_2} in response to a change in ventilation. Thus, low P_{aCO_2}, for a given metabolic rate, promotes ventilatory stability by requiring a larger increase in VE for a given reduction in arterial P_{aCO_2}, whereas high P_{aCO_2} promotes instability. Steady state hyperventilation, and hence hypocapnia, promotes stability by decreasing plant gain. The controller gain is the ventilatory response for a given change in chemical stimuli (Δ VE vs Δ P_{aCO_2}). When CSA is induced by passive mechanical hyperventilation, the controller gain represents the slope of CO_2 chemoreflex sensitivity below eupnea in response to induced hypocapnia. A high controller gain is associated with ventilatory instability, whereas a low controller gain is associated with ventilatory stability. As the blood leaves the pulmonary capillaries, the chemical stimuli are diluted by the systemic circulation and delayed by the obligatory transit time; the cerebral circulation adds further delay and dilution. Thus, P_{aCO_2} does not necessarily reflect the chemoreceptor P_{CO_2}. This point may be particularly relevant in patients with CHF and low ejection fraction who have prolonged circulation time.

Role of Central Apnea in the Development of Obstructive Sleep Apnea

A less recognized phenomenon is that CSA may also influence the development of obstructive sleep apnea (OSA) (**Fig. 1**). It has been shown that pharyngeal obstruction develops when ventilatory drive reaches a nadir during induced periodic breathing.[5,6] In studies using upper airway imaging, the authors have shown that CSA results in pharyngeal narrowing or occlusion in normal individuals and patients with sleep disordered breathing.[7,8] Patients with unfavorable upper airway anatomy may be particularly dependent on ventilatory motor output to preserve upper airway patency.[7] Pharyngeal collapse combined with mucosal and gravitational factors may impede pharyngeal opening and necessitate a substantial increase in a drive that perpetuates breathing instability.

PATHOPHYSIOLOGIC CLASSIFICATION OF CENTRAL SLEEP APNEA

The classification of CSA as hypocapnic or nonhypocapnic (based on the level of daytime P_{aCO_2}) is traditionally used. However, this classification does not capture the continuum of ventilatory abnormalities in clinical conditions.

Nonhypocapnic CSA is caused by removal of the wakefulness stimulus to breathe in patients with neuromuscular disease or severe abnormalities in pulmonary mechanics. Therefore, it is technically a form of sleep-related ventilatory failure in patients with marginal respiratory status. Hypoventilation is terminated by arousal, only to recur

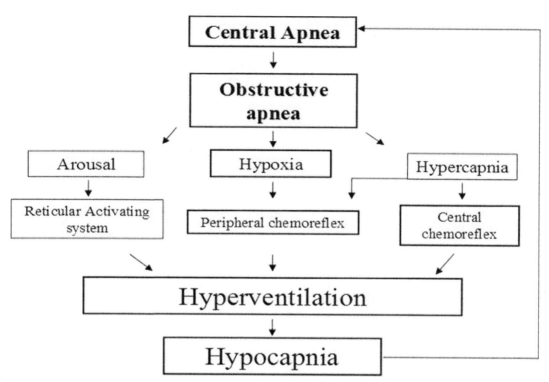

Fig. 1. Proposed mechanism by which CSAs induce obstructive apneas.

with resumption of sleep. Consequently, the presenting clinical picture includes both features of the underlying respiratory or neuromuscular disease and features of sleep apnea syndrome. This type of CSA is uncommon in patients with CHF unless a concomitant neuromuscular disease or chest wall deformity is present.

The most common underlying mechanism of CSA is hypocapnia caused by hyperventilation; this is the most relevant mechanism in patients with CHF. This type of apnea occurs in the absence of daytime alveolar hypoventilation; common features include hyperventilation and hence hypocapnia, even during wakefulness with no evidence of a comorbid respiratory conditions such as neuromuscular disorder, abnormal lung mechanics, or impaired responses to chemical stimuli. Oscillating sleep state at sleep onset or transient hypoxia (possibly caused by reduced lung volumes in obese supine patients) may trigger the first apnea, set in motion the process of apnea-hyperpnea, and lead to sustained breathing instability, manifested as periodic breathing (discussed earlier).

CENTRAL APNEA RISK FACTORS

Several physiologic or pathologic factors influence the susceptibility to, including sleep state (discussed earlier), age, gender, and several medical conditions.

The prevalence of CSA is higher in older adults compared with middle-aged adults.[9,10] The mechanisms of age-related increase in the propensity to develop CSA are multifactorial and include the increased sleep state instability that is common with aging and the increased prevalence of comorbid metabolic or cardiovascular disorders. In addition, aging may contribute to increased susceptibility to develop CSA in older adults.

CSA is uncommon in premenopausal women, who are less susceptible to hypocapnic CSA than men.[11] Manipulation of male sex hormones alters the apneic threshold in men and premenopausal women. Specifically, administration of testosterone to premenopausal women is associated with narrowing of the CO_2 reserve,[12] whereas suppression of testosterone with leuprolide acetate in healthy men is associated with widening of the CO_2 reserve.[13] In addition, menopause is associated with narrowing of the CO_2 reserve. The authors have shown that hormone replacement therapy in postmenopausal women lowers the apneic threshold and widens the CO_2 reserve to a level similar to that of premenopausal women.[14] Thus, sex hormones are important determinants of the CO_2 reserve and the apneic threshold in humans during sleep.

Sleep apnea, both obstructive and central types, has been found to be prevalent in patients with CHF.[15,16] In a group of patients referred to a sleep center, Sin and colleagues[15] found that 29% of the patients had moderate-severe CSA, whereas 32% had moderate-severe OSA. Yumino and colleagues,[17] in a study of 218 patients with CHF drawn from a cardiology clinic, found similar percentages: 26% had moderate-severe OSA and 21% had moderate-severe CSA. Important risk factors for CSA from these studies include male gender, atrial fibrillation, older age, daytime hypocapnia, diuretic use, and a larger ventilator response to carbon dioxide.[15,17,18]

Sleep apnea is common after a cerebrovascular accident (CVA), with CSA the predominant type in 40% of patients with sleep apnea following a CVA.[19–21] Likewise, CSA occurs in 30% of patients receiving stable methadone maintenance treatment[22] and has also been associated with other opioid medications (such as hydrocodone and oxycodone).[23,24] In addition, CSA occurs in several medical conditions, including hypothyroidism,[25] acromegaly,[26] and chronic renal failure.[27–29] Nocturnal hemodialysis is associated with improvement in sleep apnea indices, suggesting the important role of fluid volume and fluid shifts during sleep in the pathogenesis of CSA (also discussed later).[28]

CSA in patients with no apparent risk factor is referred to as idiopathic CSA. The only reported abnormality in these patients is increased chemoresponsiveness and sleep state instability.[30,31] However, it is unclear whether these patients have occult cardiac or metabolic disease. For instance, patients with idiopathic CSA have a higher prevalence of atrial fibrillation.[32]

MECHANISMS OF BREATHING INSTABILITY IN HEART FAILURE

Several physiologic derangements conspire to promote recurrent apnea and CSR during sleep in patients with CHF (Fig. 2). These derangements include increased peripheral and central chemoreflex sensitivity, rostral shifts of fluids, and cerebrovascular reactivity.

There is increasing evidence of the important role of the peripheral chemoreceptors (particularly the carotid bodies) in the pathophysiology of central breathing instability in patients with CHF.[33] Several studies in both humans[18,34] and animal models[35,36] of CHF have shown that carotid body chemoreceptor-mediated responses to hypoxia and hypercapnia are augmented in CHF. For instance, Giannoni and colleagues[34] found that 60% of patients with CHF had increased carotid body chemoreflex sensitivity and that patients without augmented chemosensitivity did not show CSR. In addition, deactivation (in humans)[37] or ablation (in animal models)[36] of carotid body activity results in reduction in periodic breathing. Increased chemoreflex sensitivity may further increase tonic sympathetic nervous system activity as well as modulating the phenomenon of respiratory-sympathetic coupling (in which increases in respiration are associated with increases in sympathetic activity).[33] The increased sympathetic activity, in turn, may contribute to worsened physiologic consequences of CHF,

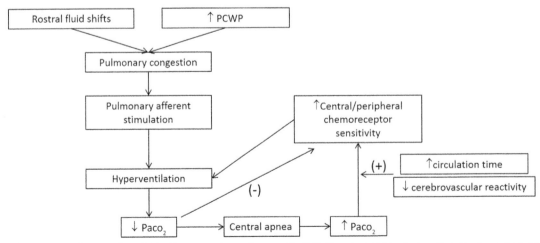

Fig. 2. The mechanisms by which CSA occurs in patients with CHF. Plus sign (+) indicates that the increased circulation time and decreased cerebrovascular reactivity delay detection of, and impair the normal buffering of, $Paco_2$ and hydrogen ion, leading to overshoot and undershoot. Minus sign (−) indicates that hypocapnia may be stabilizing by decreasing plant gain. PCWP, pulmonary capillary wedge pressure.

such as cardiorenal syndrome. High peripheral chemosensitivity has been associated with poor prognosis and higher mortality risk in patients with CHF.[38,39] However, the mechanisms by which the carotid bodies are sensitized in CHF have not been elucidated, although an association between left atrial volume and impaired chemosensitivity has been found.[40]

In addition to the role of the peripheral chemoreceptors, there is evidence of changes in the central chemoreceptor sensitivity in patients with CHF. Several groups have found that the central response to CO_2 was increased in patients with CHF.[18,41] Xie and colleagues[2] found that this increased sensitivity is associated with a narrowing of the CO_2 reserve and increased propensity to CSA.

The supine position and sleep are associated with rostral fluid shifts to the thorax; the increased fluid may stimulate ventilation by activating pulmonary stretch receptors and hypocapnia, and hence may promote ventilatory overshoot and subsequent apnea following a physiologic perturbation. This hypothesis was confirmed by Yumino and colleagues,[42] who found that larger decreases in leg fluid volume (indicating larger rostral fluid shifts) were associated with a higher CSA index and a lower transcutaneous CO_2. Pulmonary vascular congestion may also be caused by increases in the pulmonary capillary wedge pressure secondary to impaired left ventricular dysfunction; increased pulmonary capillary wedge pressure has been associated with hypocapnia and the presence of CSA.[43,44] However, although the presence of pulmonary vascular congestion in patients with CSA and CHF does lead to hyperventilation and hypocapnia,[45,46] the ensuing steady state hypocapnia could stabilize breathing by virtue of decreased plant gain; hypocapnia-associated decreased plant gain would therefore be stabilizing rather than destabilizing, as is commonly thought. Thus, the influence of rostral fluid shifts on the pathogenesis of CSA and CSR is likely mixed.

Diminished cerebrovascular reactivity to changes in $Paco_2$ is common in CHF and may further contribute to sleep-related breathing instability.[47] In this mechanism, the normal buffering action to changes in central hydrogen ion concentration is impaired, resulting in greater increase in $Paco_2$ and hydrogen ions during hypercapnia and a greater reduction during hypocapnia for a given change in $Paco_2$. Hence, the ability of the ventilator system to dampen ventilatory overshoots or undershoots is impaired.

In addition, increased circulation time secondary to decreased cardiac output may promote

further instability by delaying detection of changes in $Paco_2$ between the pulmonary capillaries and the central chemoreceptors, prolonging information feedback. Patients with systolic CHF show prolonged circulatory lung-to-ear circulation time,[48] a surrogate measure of circulatory delay and longer cycle time. Tkacova and colleagues[49] showed a shift in respiratory events during sleep from obstructive to central during the night in a group of 12 patients with CHF; the shift in respiratory events was associated with a prolongation of the circulatory time and periodic breathing cycle during the night.

SUMMARY

CSA and CSR are commonly observed breathing patterns during sleep in patients with CHF. Proposed mechanisms include augmented peripheral and central chemoreceptor sensitivity that increase ventilator instability during both wakefulness and sleep and decrease the CO_2 reserve, predisposing to sleep apnea. In addition, diminished cerebrovascular reactivity and increased circulation time impair the normal buffering of $Paco_2$ and hydrogen ions and delay the detection of changes in $Paco_2$ during sleep, leading to ventilator overshoot and undershoot. In addition, rostral fluid shifts predispose to hypocapnia, recognized as a risk factor for CSA; however, hypocapnia may also decrease plant gain, stabilizing the respiratory system. These mechanisms are likely of increased importance in older male patients with atrial fibrillation, who are at the greatest risk of developing CSA. Future research is needed to elucidate the mechanisms by which the observed changes in chemoreceptor sensitivity, CO_2 reserve, and cerebrovascular reactivity are manifested in some but not all patients with CHF, predisposing those patients to CSA and CSR.

REFERENCES

1. Skatrud JB, Dempsey JA. Interaction of sleep state and chemical stimuli in sustaining rhythmic ventilation. J Appl Physiol Respir Environ Exerc Physiol 1983;55:813–22.

2. Xie A, Skatrud JB, Puleo DS, et al. Apnea-hypopnea threshold for CO_2 in patients with congestive heart failure. Am J Respir Crit Care Med 2002;165:1245–50.

3. Orem J, Lovering AT, Dunin-Barkowski W, et al. Tonic activity in the respiratory system in wakefulness, NREM and REM sleep. Sleep 2002;25:488–96.

4. Dempsey JA, Smith CA, Przybylowski T, et al. The ventilatory responsiveness to CO(2) below eupnoea

as a determinant of ventilatory stability in sleep. J Physiol 2004;560:1–11.

5. Hudgel DW, Chapman KR, Faulks C, et al. Changes in inspiratory muscle electrical activity and upper airway resistance during periodic breathing induced by hypoxia during sleep. Am Rev Respir Dis 1987; 135:899–906.

6. Onal E, Burrows DL, Hart RH, et al. Induction of periodic breathing during sleep causes upper airway obstruction in humans. J Appl Physiol 1986;61: 1438–43.

7. Badr MS, Kawak A, Skatrud JB, et al. Effect of induced hypocapnic hypopnea on upper airway patency in humans during NREM sleep. Respir Physiol 1997;110:33–45.

8. Badr MS, Toiber F, Skatrud JB, et al. Pharyngeal narrowing/occlusion during central sleep apnea. J Appl Physiol 1995;78:1806–15.

9. Bixler EO, Vgontzas AN, Ten Have T, et al. Effects of age on sleep apnea in men: I. Prevalence and severity. Am J Respir Crit Care Med 1998;157:144–8.

10. Ancoli-Israel S, Kripke DF, Klauber MR, et al. Sleep-disordered breathing in community-dwelling elderly. Sleep 1991;14:486–95.

11. Zhou XS, Shahabuddin S, Zahn BR, et al. Effect of gender on the development of hypocapnic apnea/hypopnea during NREM sleep. J Appl Physiol 2000;89:192–9.

12. Zhou XS, Rowley JA, Demirovic F, et al. Effect of testosterone on the apneic threshold in women during NREM sleep. J Appl Physiol 2003;94:101–7.

13. Mateika JH, Omran Q, Rowley JA, et al. Treatment with leuprolide acetate decreases the threshold of the ventilatory response to carbon dioxide in healthy males. J Physiol 2004;561:637–46.

14. Rowley JA, Zhou XS, Diamond MP, et al. The determinants of the apnea threshold during NREM sleep in normal subjects. Sleep 2006;29:95–103.

15. Sin DD, Fitzgerald F, Parker JD, et al. Risk factors for central and obstructive sleep apnea in 450 men and women with congestive heart failure. Am J Respir Crit Care Med 1999;160:1101–6.

16. Javaheri S, Parker TJ, Liming JD, et al. Sleep apnea in 81 ambulatory male patients with stable heart failure. Types and their prevalences, consequences, and presentations. Circulation 1998;97:2154–9.

17. Yumino D, Wang H, Floras JS, et al. Prevalence and physiological predictors of sleep apnea in patients with heart failure and systolic dysfunction. J Card Fail 2009;15:279–85.

18. Javaheri S. A mechanism of central sleep apnea in patients with heart failure. N Engl J Med 1999;341: 949–54.

19. Parra O, Arboix A, Bechich S, et al. Time course of sleep-related breathing disorders in first-ever stroke or transient ischemic attack. Am J Respir Crit Care Med 2000;161:375–80.

20. Bassetti C, Aldrich MS. Sleep apnea in acute cerebrovascular diseases: final report on 128 patients. Sleep 1999;22:217–23.

21. Bassetti C, Aldrich MS, Chervin RD, et al. Sleep apnea in patients with transient ischemic attack and stroke: a prospective study of 59 patients. Neurology 1996;47:1167–73.

22. Wang D, Teichtahl H, Drummer O, et al. Central sleep apnea in stable methadone maintenance treatment patients. Chest 2005;128:1348–56.

23. Walker JM, Farney RJ. Are opioids associated with sleep apnea? A review of the evidence. Curr Pain Headache Rep 2009;13:120–6.

24. Walker JM, Farney RJ, Rhondeau SM, et al. Chronic opioid use is a risk factor for the development of central sleep apnea and ataxic breathing. J Clin Sleep Med 2007;3:455–61.

25. Grunstein RR, Sullivan CE. Sleep apnea and hypothyroidism: mechanisms and management. Am J Med 1988;85:775–9.

26. Grunstein RR, Ho KY, Berthon-Jones M, et al. Central sleep apnea is associated with increased ventilatory response to carbon dioxide and hypersecretion of growth hormone in patients with acromegaly. Am J Respir Crit Care Med 1994;150: 496–502.

27. Dharia SM, Unruh ML, Brown LK. Central sleep apnea in kidney disease. Semin Nephrol 2015;35: 335–46.

28. Tang SC, Lam B, Lai AS, et al. Improvement in sleep apnea during nocturnal peritoneal dialysis is associated with reduced airway congestion and better uremic clearance. Clin J Am Soc Nephrol 2009;4:410–8.

29. Fleischmann G, Fillafer G, Matterer H, et al. Prevalence of chronic kidney disease in patients with suspected sleep apnoea. Nephrol Dial Transplant 2010; 25:181–6.

30. Xie A, Rutherford R, Rankin F, et al. Hypocapnia and increased ventilatory responsiveness in patients with idiopathic central sleep apnea. Am J Respir Crit Care Med 1995;152:1950–5.

31. Xie A, Wong B, Phillipson EA, et al. Interaction of hyperventilation and arousal in the pathogenesis of idiopathic central sleep apnea. Am J Respir Crit Care Med 1994;150:489–95.

32. Leung RS, Huber MA, Rogge T, et al. Association between atrial fibrillation and central sleep apnea. Sleep 2005;28:1543–6.

33. Marcus NJ, Del Rio R, Schultz HD. Central role of carotid body chemoreceptors in disordered breathing and cardiorenal dysfunction in chronic heart failure. Front Physiol 2014;5:438.

34. Giannoni A, Emdin M, Poletti R, et al. Clinical significance of chemosensitivity in chronic heart failure: influence on neurohormonal derangement, Cheyne-Stokes respiration and arrhythmias. Clin Sci (Lond) 2008;114:489–97.

35. Haack KK, Marcus NJ, Del Rio R, et al. Simvastatin treatment attenuates increased respiratory variability and apnea/hypopnea index in rats with chronic heart failure. Hypertension 2014;63:1041–9.

36. Marcus NJ, Del Rio R, Schultz EP, et al. Carotid body denervation improves autonomic and cardiac function and attenuates disordered breathing in congestive heart failure. J Physiol 2014;592:391–408.

37. Fontana M, Emdin M, Giannoni A, et al. Effect of acetazolamide on chemosensitivity, Cheyne-Stokes respiration, and response to effort in patients with heart failure. Am J Cardiol 2011;107:1675–80.

38. Ponikowski P, Anker SD, Chua TP, et al. Oscillatory breathing patterns during wakefulness in patients with chronic heart failure: clinical implications and role of augmented peripheral chemosensitivity. Circulation 1999;100:2418–24.

39. Ponikowski P, Chua TP, Anker SD, et al. Peripheral chemoreceptor hypersensitivity: an ominous sign in patients with chronic heart failure. Circulation 2001; 104:544–9.

40. Calvin AD, Somers VK, Johnson BD, et al. Left atrial size, chemosensitivity, and central sleep apnea in heart failure. Chest 2014;146:96–103.

41. Solin P, Roebuck T, Johns DP, et al. Peripheral and central ventilatory responses in central sleep apnea with and without congestive heart failure. Am J Respir Crit Care Med 2000;162:2194–200.

42. Yumino D, Redolfi S, Ruttanaumpawan P, et al. Nocturnal rostral fluid shift: a unifying concept for the pathogenesis of obstructive and central sleep apnea in men with heart failure. Circulation 2010; 121:1598–605.

43. Solin P, Bergin P, Richardson M, et al. Influence of pulmonary capillary wedge pressure on central apnea in heart failure. Circulation 1999;99:1574–9.

44. Lorenzi-Filho G, Azevedo ER, Parker JD, et al. Relationship of carbon dioxide tension in arterial blood to pulmonary wedge pressure in heart failure. Eur Respir J 2002;19:37–40.

45. Hanly P, Zuberi N, Gray R. Pathogenesis of Cheyne-Stokes respiration in patients with congestive heart failure. Relationship to arterial PCO_2. Chest 1993; 104:1079–84.

46. Tkacova R, Hall MJ, Liu PP, et al. Left ventricular volume in patients with heart failure and Cheyne-Stokes respiration during sleep. Am J Respir Crit Care Med 1997;156:1549–55.

47. Xie A, Skatrud JB, Barczi SR, et al. Influence of cerebral blood flow on breathing stability. J Appl Physiol 2009;106:850–6.

48. Hall MJ, Xie A, Rutherford R, et al. Cycle length of periodic breathing in patients with and without heart failure. Am J Respir Crit Care Med 1996;154: 376–81.

49. Tkacova R, Niroumand M, Lorenzi-Filho G, et al. Overnight shift from obstructive to central apneas in patients with heart failure: role of PCO_2 and circulatory delay. Circulation 2001;103:238–43.

Sleep-Disordered Breathing and Arrhythmia in Heart Failure Patients

CrossMark

Henrik Fox, MD*, Thomas Bitter, MD,
Dieter Horstkotte, MD, PhD, FESC, Olaf Oldenburg, MD

KEYWORDS

- Arrhythmia • Sleep-disordered breathing (SDB) • Heart failure (HF) • Atrial fibrillation
- Sudden cardiac death

KEY POINTS

- Considering comorbidities in heart failure (HF) is important.
- Sleep-disordered breathing and arrhythmia are common in patients with HF.
- Sleep-disordered breathing and arrhythmia affect the patient's condition and prognosis, individually and through interaction.
- Sleep-disordered breathing and arrhythmia are associated with increased mortality in patients with HF.
- Treatment must consider latest research findings and outcomes.

INTRODUCTION

Despite recent strong advances in heart failure (HF) treatment, mainly in pharmacology and devices, as well as HF monitoring, patients with HF still suffer from a high burden in quality of life compromises, morbidity, and mortality.[1] Although HF is not a disease limited to the heart, rather it affects the entire organism, new approaches for understanding and improving HF are currently being studied. The recently published guideline for diagnosis and treatment of acute and chronic HF of the European Society of Cardiology focuses HF treatment not only on HF itself, but highlights the importance of attention to comorbidities in patients with HF.[1] In this context, 2 relevant and frequently observed comorbidities in patients with HF are arrhythmias and sleep-disordered breathing (SDB), both associated with morbidity and mortality[2–5] and known to worsen quality of life. Hereby, in particular, SDB is well documented to worsen quality of life, increase morbidity in general, and is clearly associated with accelerated mortality in the broad HF population.[3,4,6,7]

Patients with HF face a high risk of cardiac arrhythmias, and its clinical presentations vary from asymptomatic incidental electrocardiographic findings to palpitations and syncope, but importantly, also sudden cardiac death (SCD).[8] SDB is known to be underdiagnosed in patients with HF by far,[9] as classic symptoms are lacking in these patients and cannot be reliably determined

Conflict of interest: The authors declare that they have no conflict of interest to disclose with regard to this article.
No funding received for this article.
Clinic for Cardiology, Herz- und Diabeteszentrum NRW, Ruhr-Universität Bochum, Georgstr. 11, D-32545 Bad Oeynhausen, Germany
* Corresponding author.
E-mail address: akleemeyer@hdz-nrw.de

Sleep Med Clin 12 (2017) 229–241
http://dx.doi.org/10.1016/j.jsmc.2017.01.003
1556-407X/17/© 2017 Elsevier Inc. All rights reserved.

sleep.theclinics.com

through established questionnaires.[10] Furthermore, no biomarker exists to identify SDB,[11] whereas biomarkers have a controversial, albeit firmly established, role in HF.[1] Several population-based studies have shown an association between SDB and rhythm disorders in patients with HF.[12,13] In a recent study from Brazil, of 767 volunteers, 53.3% without SDB had cardiac rhythm disturbances, but up to 92.3% of patients with severe SDB revealed cardiac arrhythmias,[14] pointing out the importance and link of both comorbidities.[15] One of the most frequently emerging arrhythmias in cardiovascular medicine is atrial fibrillation (AF). Interestingly, it has just been published that in many cases the diagnosis of lone AF, AF without any other simultaneous disease, is false in many cases, as most studies that examined lone AF did not test for SDB. This suggests that many patients with lone AF have undiagnosed SDB.[16]

As the item-centered view extends HF and includes comorbidities now, such as the aforementioned, numerous questions arise not only on their characteristics and therapy alone, but also about their connection and therapy implications.

HEART FAILURE AND ARRHYTHMIA

HF is a major health care concern in modern medicine, as the number of patients suffering from HF is actually rising.[1] The exact prevalence of HF varies in different publications, as the definition of HF is inconsistent and deviates among the different societies.[1,17,18] Depending on the definition used, HF prevalence is approximately 1% to 2% of the adult population in developed countries,[1,17,18] quickly rising to more than 10% among patients older than 70.[1,17–20] In HF, 2 major types need to be distinguished: HF with reduced ejection fraction (HFrEF) and HF with preserved ejection fraction (HFpEF).[1,17,18] The European Society of Cardiology recently introduced a third term, HF with mid-range ejection fraction, to allow more clarification in these in-between patients.[1] Prognosis of patients with HF is still poor,[21] and for patients older than 65 presenting to their doctor for breathlessness on exertion, 1 in 6 will have unrecognized HF, mainly HFpEF.[1,22] Unison among all definitions, HF remains a clinical diagnosis with the symptoms in focus,[1] bearing in mind that typical symptoms and signs of HF due to fluid retention may quickly resolve with diuretic therapy.[1] Signs, such as elevated jugular venous pressure and displacement of the apical impulse, are more specific, but are harder to detect, especially in obese and elderly patients, or patients with chronic lung disease,[1] which makes taking a

detailed history and obtaining comprehensive clinical examination absolutely essential.

Appearance of arrhythmias is frequent in patients with HF and it denotes an increase in mortality.[8] Although different types of arrhythmias, such as AF, atrial flutter, ventricular tachycardia, but also bradycardias and pauses, all contribute to deterioration in quality of life, increased hospitalization rates, and augmented mortality,[8] their entity, combination, and characteristics are to be considered in the context of the underlying cardiac disease and the stage of HF.[1] Although the lifetime risk of developing HF at an age of 55 years is 33% for men and 28% for women,[20] nearly every patient is found to have some sort of arrhythmia,[1] and arrhythmia can contribute to not only lower quality of life but also increased symptoms of HF.[1]

LINK BETWEEN SLEEP-DISORDERED BREATHING AND CARDIAC ARRHYTHMIA IN HEART FAILURE

Both SDB and arrhythmia have a high prevalence in patients with HF.[1,9] Broad registries have identified a prevalence of moderate to severe SDB in patients with HF of more than 50%[9,23] and with the numbers of comorbidities increasing, SDB prevalence reaches a percentage of more than 90%.[15] In addition, cardiac arrhythmias are highly common in patients with HF.[1] Through long-term electrocardiographic recordings, premature ventricular complexes are found in nearly every patient with HF,[1] and episodes of asymptomatic, nonsustained ventricular tachycardia are common, increasing in frequency with HF severity and left ventricular dysfunction.[1] Moreover bradycardia and pauses are also frequently found, with those episodes predominantly occurring during night hours when sympathetic activity is lowered and parasympathetic activity is increased,[1] which makes underlying diseases such as SDB ominous. In this regard, the link between SDB and cardiac arrhythmias was impressively demonstrated in the DREAM study, in which compared with patients without SDB, patients with moderate to severe SDB had an almost threefold unadjusted odds of any cardiac arrhythmia.[24] In this study, a cross-sectional analysis of 697 veterans who underwent polysomnography,[24] patients with SDB still had twice the odds of having nocturnal cardiac arrhythmias even after adjustment for age, body mass index, gender, and cardiovascular disease, with the frequency of obstructive respiratory events and hypoxia predicting arrhythmia risk.[24]

In this context, the recently published guideline for diagnosis and treatment of acute and chronic HF of the European Society of Cardiology and others state that sleep apnea may be a trigger.[1,25] Moreover, the recently released guidelines of the task force for the European Society of Cardiology for management of AF implement SDB as a condition independently associated with AF.[26,27] SDB also is especially mentioned and highlighted in the American Heart Association (AHA)/American College of Cardiology/Heart Rhythm Society guideline for the management of AF,[28] the American College of Cardiology Foundation/AHA guideline for HF,[17] and in many other recommendation articles, like the Japanese Cardiac Society HF guidelines.[18]

Interestingly, the diagnosis of SDB in patients with HF cannot be assisted with the help of biomarkers, which are fairly established in HF.[11] Attempts to simplify SDB diagnosis in patients with HF with the use of biomarkers failed, which leaves many patients with HF and arrhythmia undiagnosed and subsequently untreated for SDB.[11] Nevertheless, pretest probability for presence of SDB is high in patients with HF and arrhythmia and even increases with age, as age is a robust risk factor for SDB.[29]

With these 2 comorbidities, SDB and cardiac arrhythmia, in focus, over the recent years several studies identified SDB to be an important factor in arrhythmogenesis and questions arise whether SDB treatment may lower cardiac arrhythmia burden and even have the potential to improve quality of life, morbidity, and mortality.

INTERPLAY OF SDB AND CARDIAC ARRHYTHMIA: PATHOPHYSIOLOGY AND AUTONOMIC TONE

With adults spending more than two-thirds of total sleep time in non–rapid eye movement sleep, these sleep stages are considered to be of predominant parasympathetic tone and hence reduced sympathetic neural activity.[30,31] Recent studies that explain the interaction of SDB and arrhythmia have identified nocturnal hypoxemia to be a relevant trigger of cardiac arrhythmias.[5,32] Thereby, nocturnal hypoxemia and hypercapnia are associated with increased sympathetic nervous system activity, which fragment regular nightly sleep and lead to the usual complaints of patients with SDB, such as sleepiness, fatigue, and poor concentration abilities.[33] Whether late risers or short-time sleepers have a different arrhythmia burden is unknown, but sleep stages and neural activity are well understood and widely studied outliers in SDB pathophysiology and they are equivocally linked to be a trigger for cardiac arrhythmias.[30] In addition, it has been demonstrated before that negative intrathoracic pressure

changes trigger arrhythmias, such as AF, also by shortening effective atrial refractory periods, which is mainly due to enhanced vagal activation.[34] On the other hand, bradyarrhythmias are linked to vagal activation, which was identified at the end of apneic events, and vagal activation is mediated by hypoxemic triggering of the glomus caroticum.[35] During these disturbances of nerve activity and intrabody pressures, SDB is further known to be associated with surges in blood pressure and heart rate. In turn, they enhance myocardial oxygen demand and cardiac workload and explain why SDB makes the heart more vulnerable to arrhythmias during nightly hours.[36]

Autonomic neural inputs to ganglionated plexi and resulting enhanced ganglionated plexus activity is illustrated to be associated with this shortening of atrial refractory periods, promoting premature and odd stimuli of myocardial activity, best studied for atrial myocardial activation.[30,32,37] Ghias and colleagues[38] found after neural ablation of ganglionated plexi that inducibility of AF was significantly lower and in this relationship renal denervation was demonstrated to reduce shortening of atrial effective refractory periods in an animal model of obstructive SDB,[39] underlining the present pathophysiologic understanding, while decided details on neural activity are still under investigation.[38,39]

SLEEP-DISORDERED BREATHING PATHOPHYSIOLOGY AND SYSTEMIC CARDIOVASCULAR EFFECTS

Negative intrathoracic pressures and distension on the vessels have been associated in SDB with vasodilation,[15] but SDB does not only promote local vasodilating effects, because apneas have been found to be associated with systemic vasoconstriction as well. This vasoconstriction again can increase cardiac afterload, cardiac workload, and myocardial oxygen demand.[40] In addition, intrathoracic pressure changes and hypoxemia-induced vasoconstriction increase shear stress, and chronic shear stress can lead to myocardial remodeling and HF advance.[41,42] Derangements in hormone activity in SDB include increased plasma renin activity and aldosterone concentrations in obstructive SDB. In a pig model, reproducing obstructive SDB episodes using exposure to repetitive obstructive respiratory events for 4 hours, resulted in an increased expression of connective tissue growth factor, a redox-sensitive mediator of fibrosis.[39] However, with regard to the renin-angiotensin-aldosterone system, a major driver of hypertension and cardiovascular disease, little evidence supports the association of

SDB with increased levels of angiotensin II and aldosterone in humans.[43,44] SDB with intermittent hypoxemia during repetitive airflow cessations also can lead to endothelial dysfunction. SDB also has been shown to be associated with many other impacts, such as hypercoagulability, decreased nitric oxide levels, impaired vasodilation, increased systemic inflammation, sympathetic nervous system activation, increased oxidative stress, and dysglycemia, which may all contribute to cardiovascular diseases, such as hypertension, stroke, and coronary artery disease, adding to HF and arrhythmia.[45,46] Although the development of cardiovascular disease seems favored in the presence of SDB, and yet cardiovascular disease predisposes to cardiac arrhythmia,[46] plurality of factors come into play (Fig. 1). In this context, SDB has been shown to lead and assess at multiple starting points, adding reduction in the atrial effective refractory period, triggered and abnormal automaticity, and promote slowed and heterogeneous conduction, mechanisms that increase the persistence of re-entrant arrhythmias, and prolong the QT interval.[46] With this complex interplay, numerous questions are still unanswered and demand further investigation.

SLEEP-DISORDERED BREATHING AND ATRIAL FIBRILLATION

When it comes to atrial arrhythmias, AF and atrial flutter are the entities of major clinical importance,[1,16] with the prevalence of AF and atrial flutter among patients with HF being high.[1] Adding to this, the prevalence of SDB among patients with AF or atrial flutter also is high.[47–50] Nevertheless, no single line of connection between these diseases can be drawn, as both diseases share common cardiovascular risk factors, such as hypertension or obesity.[30,51,52] An increasing incidence of AF in large cohort studies in patients with

obstructive SDB is nicely documented,[26] and even in specific patient cohorts, such as patients with hypertrophic cardiomyopathy, obstructive SDB is independently associated with an increased risk of AF onset.[53] Adding to this, not only obstructive sleep apnea (OSA) has been shown to increase the risk for AF, but also central SDB and Cheyne-Stokes respiration (CSR) have clearly been illustrated to predict incident AF in the MrOS Sleep study.[54] Therein, in a cohort of 843 men without prevalent AF, central sleep apnea (CSA) and CSR predicted incident AF.[54]

Notably, identification of SDB in patients with AF is challenging and requires simple device-based screening, because SDB questionnaires are not specific for AF and have never been validated in patients with AF.[55] Even more accurately, studies found no association between the Epworth Sleepiness Scale[56] score and the severity of SDB in these patients,[55] which makes the standard approach of basic questions for SDB identification in these patients defective[10,55] and points out that established and easily deployable technical examinations are necessary for screening as recommended.[57] Explanations assumed to this circumstance, include that AF per se is associated with poor sleep quality, which makes identification of the additional comorbidity of SDB difficult.[58]

SLEEP-DISORDERED BREATHING AND ATRIAL FIBRILLATION: PATHOPHYSIOLOGY

Apneas and hypopneas of SDB are often associated with excessive negative intrathoracic pressure changes that alter transmural pressures and cardiac and vessel volume relations[30,59] (Fig. 2). SDB is believed to promote cardiac and, in particular, atrial remodeling. In an animal model, Iwasaki and colleagues[60] were able to demonstrate obstructive SDB to cause left ventricular hypertrophy, ventricular dilation, and diastolic dysfunction,

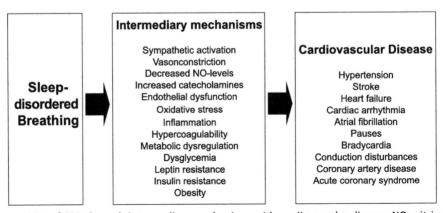

Fig. 1. Connectivity of SDB through intermediary mechanisms with cardiovascular disease. NO, nitric oxide.

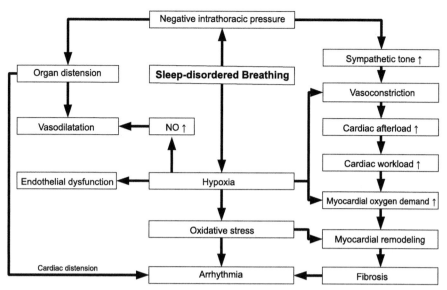

Fig. 2. Interplay and connectivity of SDB with manifold cardiovascular effects and links. NO, nitric oxide.

as well as a connexin dysregulation and an increase in atrial fibrous tissue burden. Additionally, these transformations were explicitly associated with enhanced inducibility of AF.[60] In a small study of 40 patients undergoing catheter ablation for paroxysmal AF, obstructive SDB was also associated with increased atrial remodeling and reduced myocardial voltage, as well as site-specific and widespread myocardial conduction disturbances.[30,61] With these alterations in the heart, subsequent, nocturnal distensions to the atrium through SDB may be an important trigger for the onset of AF in patients with HF with SDB.[47,62] Correspondingly, several studies found more left atrium dilatation in patients with obstructive SDB and more impaired left atrial function compared with control subjects without SDB[41,63] (**Fig. 3**). Another well-established factor for cardiac remodeling is inflammation. Recent data revealed both obstructive and central SDB to be associated with enhanced inflammation,[64,65] with more studies in this field to come.

SLEEP-DISORDERED BREATHING AND ATRIAL FIBRILLATION: TREATMENT OF ATRIAL FIBRILLATION

It has been demonstrated that nonresponders to antiarrhythmic drug treatment with AF reoccurrence are more likely to have severe obstructive SDB than those without (52% vs 23%).[66] Moreover, it has been shown that the recurrence of AF after external, electric cardioversion at 12 months was 82% in patients with untreated obstructive SDB compared with 53% in patients who were not tested for SDB,[67] whereas after cardioversion it has been shown that the characteristics of SDB may even change.[47] In addition, current AF management guidelines[27,28] mention SDB as being closely associated with AF and as a factor contributing to a reduced success of ablation procedures and appeal for SDB screening.[27,28]

With the numbers of invasive catheter-based procedures rising to find a remedy for AF, our group conducted a study revealing SDB to have a negative effect on sinus rhythm persistence after a cryo-balloon ablation procedure.[68] Analog data have been published with regard to other ablation techniques, such as radiofrequency ablation for AF or cavotricuspid isthmus radiofrequency ablation for atrial flutter.[30,50,69,70]

SLEEP-DISORDERED BREATHING AND ATRIAL FIBRILLATION: TREATMENT OF SLEEP-DISORDERED BREATHING

Nocturnal continuous positive airway pressure (CPAP) therapy is the treatment of choice for

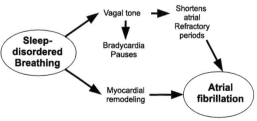

Fig. 3. Interplay and connectivity of SDB with AF and associated factors.

obstructive SDB, greatly achieving effective suppression of respiratory events. There are clues that CPAP therapy might favorably influence AF in patients with obstructive SDB, regarding sinus rhythm maintenance, that is, after AF catheter ablation[69,70] or after external, electrical cardioversion.[67] There even have been case reports that CPAP therapy alone could reverse AF back into sinus rhythm,[71] which will need further exploration. Freedom from obstructive respiratory events in patients with OSA by using CPAP reduces the risk of AF recurrence after ablation therapy.[72] CPAP therapy in patients with OSA and AF undergoing pulmonary vein isolation was associated with a higher AF-free survival rate (71.9% vs 36.7% in untreated patients)[70] and was almost similar to a group of patients without OSA.[70] Interestingly, the effect of CPAP in patients without pulmonary vein ablation was comparable to the effect of pulmonary vein isolation in CPAP non-user patients with OSA.[70] The proportion of patients who were free of AF without drug treatment or repeated ablation was also significantly higher in CPAP users versus non-CPAP users.[70]

With high expectations in this field, results from an ongoing Norwegian study are awaited, prospectively investigating 100 patients with paroxysmal AF and with moderate to severe SDB (Apnea Hypopnea Index [AHI] >15/h), that are randomized 1:1 to CPAP or control after subcutaneous implantation of an event recorder to capture AF burden with and without CPAP therapy (ClinicalTrials.gov Identifier: NCT02727192).

SLEEP-DISORDERED BREATHING AND SUDDEN CARDIAC DEATH

Events of SCD are unusual to occur during nighttime in the general population,[73] which is in contrast to what was found in patients with mainly obstructive SDB.[74] Particularly in patients with OSA, the peak of an SCD event was observed during sleeping hours,[74] data which were collected in a large population of 10,701 adults followed for 15 years.[74,75] Thereby, OSA was identified to be an independent risk factor for an SCD incident,[74,75] with a risk prediction by various SDB parameters and its severity, including nocturnal hypoxemia[5,74,75] (**Fig. 4**). Moreover, in patients with an already high risk of SCD, not only because of cardiovascular disease, but with Brugada syndrome or hypertrophic cardiomyopathy, or in implantable cardioverter-defibrillator (ICD) recipients, the prevalence of SDB was found to be high, which is believed to have the potential to even accelerate the risk for an SCD event.[76–79]

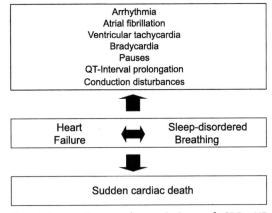

Fig. 4. Interactions and associations of SDB, HF, arrhythmia, and SCD. QT interval represents electrical depolarization and repolarization of the ventricles.

In this context, not only declined systolic and diastolic left ventricular function was found during respiratory events in patients with obstructive SDB,[59,80] but SDB has been shown to affect cardiac electrophysiology by modifying conduction velocity and refractoriness, as it has been demonstrated that obstructive SDB is associated with prolongation of the corrected QT interval and corrected T-peak to T-end interval and the TpTe/QT ratio.[81] In addition, obstructive SDB affects QT dispersion and T-wave alternans, a condition that might promote malignant arrhythmias and even SCD.[82–85] Furthermore, an AHI equal to or more than 20/h was identified as a significant and independent risk factor for an incident of SCD in a study of more than 10,000 patients examined with polysomnography.[75] Regarding arrhythmia, also the aforementioned intermittent hypoxemia and increased sympathetic nerve system activity are closely related to SDB and are associated with occurrence of premature ventricular beats.[32,86]

SLEEP-DISORDERED BREATHING AND VENTRICULAR ARRHYTHMIA

Cardiac arrhythmias, such as sustained ventricular tachyarrhythmias, are life-threatening events with major prognostic impact in patients with HF.[1] Suffering from both HF and SDB increases the risk of developing malignant ventricular arrhythmias.[87] Severe OSA increases the risk of ventricular premature beats, nonsustained and sustained ventricular tachycardia, and may contribute to nocturnal SCD.[74,88] The likelihood of AF and/or ventricular tachycardia episodes to occur was 18 times higher within a 90-second time relationship to an appearance of an apnea or a hypopnea compared with patterns with normal breathing.[89] Registry data and data from a randomized controlled trial (RCT) show that treatment of central SDB, and in particular CSR with adaptive servoventilation (ASV) therapy in patients with HF with ICD devices, reduces the necessary response of defibrillatory therapies, and improves cardiac function as well as respiratory stability.[90,91]

In focus as a high risk of developing malignant arrhythmic events are patients with chronic HF (CHF).[1] Recent data suggest a close association between development or even triggering of ventricular arrhythmias and the presence of SDB, especially in patients with CHF.[92–94] As all currently used ICD systems automatically store intracardiac electrogram recordings, an association between SDB and life-threatening arrhythmias can be easily determined.[95] Hereby, when SDB is present, more ICD therapies are found in patients with CHF compared with those without concomitant SDB.[95] In even more advanced cardiac device therapies, such as cardiac resynchronization devices, including a defibrillator, we discovered in 255 patients screened for SDB 6 months after implantation, that in 75 patients, appropriate defibrillator therapies during a 48-month follow-up period resulted in an independent association between SDB and life-threatening ventricular arrhythmia.[87] However, the literature in this field is heterogeneous to the present day.[77,96] Although some studies supported our finding and identified SDB as a risk factor for malignant arrhythmic events,[96] a study by Grimm and colleagues did not.[77] Besides these data, the resulting discrepancy may be explained by the different patient selection criteria used in the differing studies.[77,96]

In addition, cardiac device recipients are in relevant risk to be affected by inappropriate shocks as well; for instance, for false detected supraventricular arrhythmias, such as sinus tachycardias.[97] Inappropriate shocks also can result from technical issues within the device or the cords,[97] but whatever cause results in an inappropriate shock, they connote psychological consequences, reduce quality of life, and are also associated with an impaired prognosis in those patients.[97,98] To connect these dots, and because of the commonness of supraventricular arrhythmias as a major contributor to inappropriate shock device therapies, we conducted a study investigating the relation of such events to SDB.[99] Likely, because of a low rate of ICD shocks observed during follow-up, no link in this context could be portrayed yet.[99]

SLEEP-DISORDERED BREATHING AND CONDUCTION DISTURBANCES

SDB is not only associated with atrial and ventricular arrhythmias, but several smaller studies have argued an association between SDB and conduction disturbances of the heart as well.[100–102] Not only did these studies show an association of SDB and conduction disturbances, but there is also literature suggesting the potential of reducing these arrhythmia events through initiation of CPAP therapy.[101,103–105] Surprisingly in a large observational cohort study, the "Outcome of Sleep Disorders in Older Men or in the Sleep Heart Health study," no such association between SDB and heart block or bradycardias were found significantly.[12,88]

SLEEP-DISORDERED BREATHING AND ARRHYTHMIA DAYTIME DISTRIBUTION

Looking at the daytime when cardiac arrhythmias typically occur or when they are to be expected, one has to distinguish between the effects of the 2 major different types of SDB (OSA vs CSA) on circadian arrhythmia distribution in patients with CHF.[30,94] OSA has a typical peak of appropriate defibrillator shocks during the night and sleeping hours, as is to be expected through its pathophysiology,[106] but in patients with CSA, no assignment to any circadian distribution of arrhythmic events was found.[106]

IMPROVING HEART FAILURE AND ARRHYTHMIA BURDEN OUTCOME WITH SLEEP-DISORDERED BREATHING TREATMENT? WHAT IS THE EVIDENCE?

Overall, data supporting a reduction of malignant arrhythmic events, improving cardiovascular mortality, or reducing hospitalization for worsening of HF through positive airway pressure treatment are lacking. Results of the recent large RCT, the SERVE HF trial, showed fewer numbers of shocks through implanted cardiac devices in 1325 prospectively investigated patients, but treatment with adaptive servoventilation for central SDB in patients with systolic HF came with a 28% increase in all-cause mortality and 34% increased cardiovascular mortality.[91] Identification of reasons for this increased mortality through adaptive servoventilation therapy is still ongoing,[107,108] but since this trial was presented, ASV therapy for predominantly central SDB in patients with systolic HF is now clearly contraindicated.[1] On the other hand, the recently presented SAFE trial in fact missed its primary endpoint for CPAP to reduce cardiovascular events in obstructive SDB in 2717 patients. In that trial, numerous secondary endpoints for cardiovascular outcomes, such as health-related quality of life, snoring symptoms, daytime sleepiness, mood, and days absent at work for illness, could be improved.[109] Interpretation of the SAFE trial results need to include factors, such as that patients with symptomatic, severe obstructive SDB were excluded, there was low adherence to CPAP therapy, and there were overall low event rates.

Uncertainties regarding the impact of high pressures with positive airway pressures, to affect intrathoracic pressures as an explanation for these findings and the increased death rates in SERVE HF, could recently be ruled out,[107] still leaving the question of possible alternative therapies.[108] In addition, for both obstructive SDB and central SDB, device-based therapies are available and have proven safety and efficacy,[110–113] but proof of benefit in cardiovascular outcomes with these alternative therapies have not been demonstrated yet.

Therefore, the impact of SDB therapy for hard clinical endpoints, such as mortality, remains unclear to date, although recent data show in patients with preserved left ventricular ejection fraction may be in favor through ASV therapy treatment for a combined endpoint in a very recent randomized controlled clinical trial.[114]

Future, large, prospective RCTs are essential to further investigate the effect of any SDB therapy on cardiac arrhythmia and clinical endpoints in patients with HF.

IS HFPEF DIFFERENT WITH REGARD TO SDB?

Most data available on SDB and HF and most patient studies in this regard are patients with HF with reduced left ventricular systolic ejection fraction. In terms of patients with HFpEF, only a few data are available, and the association of SDB, HF, and arrhythmia in HFpEF is far less investigated yet, leaving the impact of SDB and arrhythmia unclear in this group. The prevalence of SDB has also shown to be high,[115] but challenges like HFpEF diagnosis has recently brought the European Society of Cardiology to more clearly define HFpEF diagnosis in their guideline.[1] Nevertheless, there is evidence of an association of HFpEF, SDB, and arrhythmia, with SDB being a potential target of treatment in HFpEF as well. We investigated 60 patients with HFpEF with CSR and treated with adaptive servoventilation positive airway therapy and we found significantly positive effects in absolute and predicted peak oxygen consumption, oxygen consumption at the individual aerobic-anaerobic threshold, oxygen pulse, as well as left atrial size, and transmitral flow patterns through therapy initiation.[116] Furthermore, there are ongoing studies in this field, which will elucidate therapy options for patients with HFpEF in the near future (Positive Airway Pressure Therapy Study in Sleep Apnea and Diastolic Heart Failure [Paradise HF], NCT02254382).

SUMMARY AND OUTLOOK

SDB plays an active, tight and important role in HF, and through its pathophysiology, such as myocardial remodeling processes, SDB is identified to be a trigger of arrhythmic events and SDB was related to be a significant risk factor for cardiovascular disease. In the interaction among HF, SDB, and cardiac arrhythmia, the interplay has relevant impact on quality of life, morbidity, and mortality in patients with HF. Therefore, SDB is a target in primary and secondary cardiovascular prevention, leaving most current patients undiagnosed. The latest results of large clinical trials question the current established therapy approach, as nocturnal positive airway pressure ventilation treatment of SDB seems not to be suitable for every patient with HF. Nevertheless, SDB treatment appears to be requested and desired, and therapy has been shown to beneficially influence and reduce occurrence and recurrence of cardiac arrhythmic events, especially when it comes to AF. However, a solid proof of benefits in survival in patients with HF through SDB treatment has not been demonstrated yet. In this context, many more studies are presently on their way and with great interest the results of large, prospective, clinical, controlled, randomized trials, such as the "Effect of Adaptive Servo Ventilation (ASV) on Survival and Hospital Admissions in Heart Failure (ADVENT-HF)," ClinicalTrials.gov Identifier: NCT01128816, are awaited, as the various open questions in the field of SDB, HF, and cardiac arrhythmias can be answered only through further efforts in research and realization of large trials to not only achieve clarity in treatment indications, but most importantly facilitate benefits in the treatment strategies of our patients with HF.

REFERENCES

1. Ponikowski P, Voors AA, Anker SD, et al. 2016 ESC guidelines for the diagnosis and treatment of acute and chronic heart failure: the Task Force for the diagnosis and treatment of acute and chronic heart failure of the European Society of Cardiology (ESC) developed with the special contribution of the Heart Failure Association (HFA) of the ESC. Eur Heart J 2016;37(27):2129–200.
2. Bloch Thomsen PE, Jons C, Raatikainen MJ, et al. Long-term recording of cardiac arrhythmias with an implantable cardiac monitor in patients with reduced ejection fraction after acute myocardial

infarction: the Cardiac Arrhythmias and Risk Stratification after Acute Myocardial Infarction (CARISMA) study. Circulation 2010;122(13):1258–64.

3. Jilek C, Krenn M, Sebah D, et al. Prognostic impact of sleep disordered breathing and its treatment in heart failure: an observational study. Eur J Heart Fail 2011;13(1):68–75.

4. Javaheri S, Shukla R, Zeigler H, et al. Central sleep apnea, right ventricular dysfunction, and low diastolic blood pressure are predictors of mortality in systolic heart failure. J Am Coll Cardiol 2007; 49(20):2028–34.

5. Oldenburg O, Wellmann B, Buchholz A, et al. Nocturnal hypoxaemia is associated with increased mortality in stable heart failure patients. Eur Heart J 2016;37(21):1695–703.

6. Khayat R, Jarjoura D, Porter K, et al. Sleep disordered breathing and post-discharge mortality in patients with acute heart failure. Eur Heart J 2015;36(23):1463–9.

7. Oldenburg O, Bitter T, Fox H, et al. Heart failure. Somnologie - Schlafforschung und Schlafmedizin 2014;18(1):19–25.

8. Boehmer JP, Carlson MD, De Marco T, et al. Adjudication of mortality events in a heart failure-arrhythmia trial by a multiparameter descriptive method: comparison with methods used in heart failure trials and methods used in arrhythmia trials. J Interv Card Electrophysiol 2008;23(2):101–10.

9. Arzt M, Woehrle H, Oldenburg O, et al. Prevalence and predictors of sleep-disordered breathing in patients with stable chronic heart failure: the SchlaHF registry. JACC Heart Fail 2016;4(2): 116–25.

10. Bitter T, Westerheide N, Hossain SM, et al. Symptoms of sleep apnoea in chronic heart failure–results from a prospective cohort study in 1,500 patients. Sleep Breath 2012;16(3):781–91.

11. Maeder MT, Mueller C, Schoch OD, et al. Biomarkers of cardiovascular stress in obstructive sleep apnea. Clin Chim Acta 2016;460:152–63.

12. Mehra R, Stone KL, Varosy PD, et al. Nocturnal arrhythmias across a spectrum of obstructive and central sleep-disordered breathing in older men: outcomes of sleep disorders in older men (MrOS sleep) study. Arch Intern Med 2009;169(12): 1147–55.

13. Namtvedt SK, Randby A, Einvik G, et al. Cardiac arrhythmias in obstructive sleep apnea (from the Akershus sleep apnea project). Am J Cardiol 2011;108(8):1141–6.

14. Cintra FD, Leite RP, Storti LJ, et al. Sleep apnea and nocturnal cardiac arrhythmia: a populational study. Arq Bras Cardiol 2014;103(5):368–74.

15. Linz D, Woehrle H, Bitter T, et al. The importance of sleep-disordered breathing in cardiovascular disease. Clin Res Cardiol 2015;104(9):705–18.

16. Camm AJ, Savelieva I, Potpara T, et al. The changing circumstance of atrial fibrillation—progress towards precision medicine. J Intern Med 2016; 279(5):412–27.

17. Yancy CW, Jessup M, Bozkurt B, et al. 2013 ACCF/ AHA guideline for the management of heart failure: a report of the American College of Cardiology Foundation/American Heart Association task force on practice guidelines. J Am Coll Cardiol 2013; 62(16):e147–239.

18. JCS Joint Working Group. Guidelines for treatment of acute heart failure (JCS 2011). Circ J 2013;77(8): 2157–201.

19. Mosterd A, Hoes AW. Clinical epidemiology of heart failure. Heart 2007;93(9):1137–46.

20. Bleumink GS, Knetsch AM, Sturkenboom MC, et al. Quantifying the heart failure epidemic: prevalence, incidence rate, lifetime risk and prognosis of heart failure The Rotterdam Study. Eur Heart J 2004; 25(18):1614–9.

21. Meta-analysis Global Group in Chronic Heart Failure (MAGGIC). The survival of patients with heart failure with preserved or reduced left ventricular ejection fraction: an individual patient data meta-analysis. Eur Heart J 2012;33(14):1750–7.

22. van Riet EE, Hoes AW, Limburg A, et al. Prevalence of unrecognized heart failure in older persons with shortness of breath on exertion. Eur J Heart Fail 2014;16(7):772–7.

23. Oldenburg O, Lamp B, Faber L, et al. Sleep-disordered breathing in patients with symptomatic heart failure: a contemporary study of prevalence in and characteristics of 700 patients. Eur J Heart Fail 2007;9(3):251–7.

24. Selim BJ, Koo BB, Qin L, et al. The association between nocturnal cardiac arrhythmias and sleep-disordered breathing: the DREAM study. J Clin Sleep Med 2016;12(6):829–37.

25. Gilat H, Vinker S, Buda I, et al. Obstructive sleep apnea and cardiovascular comorbidities: a large epidemiologic study. Medicine (Baltimore) 2014; 93(9):e45.

26. Gami AS, Hodge DO, Herges RM, et al. Obstructive sleep apnea, obesity, and the risk of incident atrial fibrillation. J Am Coll Cardiol 2007;49(5): 565–71.

27. Kirchhof P, Benussi S, Kotecha D, et al. 2016 ESC guidelines for the management of atrial fibrillation developed in collaboration with EACTS: the task force for the management of atrial fibrillation of the European Society of Cardiology (ESC) developed with the special contribution of the European Heart Rhythm Association (EHRA) of the ESC endorsed by the European Stroke Organisation (ESO). Eur Heart J 2016;37(38):2893–962.

28. January CT, Wann LS, Alpert JS, et al. 2014 AHA/ ACC/HRS guideline for the management of

patients with atrial fibrillation: a report of the American College of Cardiology/American Heart Association task force on practice guidelines and the Heart Rhythm Society. J Am Coll Cardiol 2014; 64(21):e1–76.

29. Morrell MJ, McMillan A. Does age Matter? The relationship between sleep-disordered breathing and incident atrial fibrillation in older men. Am J Respir Crit Care Med 2016;193(7):712–4.

30. Bitter T, Fox H, Gaddam S, et al. Sleep-disordered breathing and cardiac arrhythmias. Can J Cardiol 2015;31(7):928–34.

31. Trinder J, Kleiman J, Carrington M, et al. Autonomic activity during human sleep as a function of time and sleep stage. J Sleep Res 2001;10(4):253–64.

32. Solin P, Kaye DM, Little PJ, et al. Impact of sleep apnea on sympathetic nervous system activity in heart failure. Chest 2003;123(4):1119–26.

33. Berry RB, Budhiraja R, Gottlieb DJ, et al. Rules for scoring respiratory events in sleep: update of the 2007 AASM Manual for the scoring of sleep and associated events. Deliberations of the sleep apnea definitions task force of the American Academy of Sleep Medicine. J Clin Sleep Med 2012; 8(5):597–619.

34. Linz D, Schotten U, Neuberger HR, et al. Negative tracheal pressure during obstructive respiratory events promotes atrial fibrillation by vagal activation. Heart Rhythm 2011;8(9):1436–43.

35. Guilleminault C, Connolly S, Winkle R, et al. Cyclical variation of the heart rate in sleep apnea syndrome. Mechanisms, and usefulness of 24 h electrocardiography as a screening technique. Lancet 1984;1(8369):126–31.

36. Linz D, Mahfoud F, Schotten U, et al. Renal sympathetic denervation suppresses postapneic blood pressure rises and atrial fibrillation in a model for sleep apnea. Hypertension 2012;60(1):172–8.

37. Stevenson IH, Roberts-Thomson KC, Kistler PM, et al. Atrial electrophysiology is altered by acute hypercapnia but not hypoxemia: implications for promotion of atrial fibrillation in pulmonary disease and sleep apnea. Heart Rhythm 2010;7(9): 1263–70.

38. Ghias M, Scherlag BJ, Lu Z, et al. The role of ganglionated plexi in apnea-related atrial fibrillation. J Am Coll Cardiol 2009;54(22):2075–83.

39. Linz D, Hohl M, Nickel A, et al. Effect of renal denervation on neurohumoral activation triggering atrial fibrillation in obstructive sleep apnea. Hypertension 2013;62(4):767–74.

40. Fletcher EC. Effect of episodic hypoxia on sympathetic activity and blood pressure. Respir Physiol 2000;119(2–3):189–97.

41. Oliveira W, Campos O, Bezerra Lira-Filho E, et al. Left atrial volume and function in patients with obstructive sleep apnea assessed by real-time three-dimensional echocardiography. J Am Soc Echocardiogr 2008;21(12):1355–61.

42. Bitter T, Horstkotte D, Oldenburg O. Sleep disordered breathing and cardiac arrhythmias: mechanisms, interactions, and clinical relevance. Dtsch Med Wochenschr 2011;136(9):431–5 [in German].

43. Pratt-Ubunama MN, Nishizaka MK, Boedefeld RL, et al. Plasma aldosterone is related to severity of obstructive sleep apnea in subjects with resistant hypertension. Chest 2007;131(2):453–9.

44. Moller DS, Lind P, Strunge B, et al. Abnormal vasoactive hormones and 24-hour blood pressure in obstructive sleep apnea. Am J Hypertens 2003; 16(4):274–80.

45. Uyar M, Davutoglu V. An update on cardiovascular effects of obstructive sleep apnoea syndrome. Postgrad Med J 2016;92(1091):540–4.

46. May AM, Van Wagoner DR, Mehra R. Obstructive sleep apnea and cardiac arrhythmogenesis: Mechanistic insights. Chest 2017;151(1):225–41.

47. Fox H, Bitter T, Horstkotte D, et al. Cardioversion of atrial fibrillation or atrial flutter into sinus rhythm reduces nocturnal central respiratory events and unmasks obstructive sleep apnoea. Clin Res Cardiol 2016;105(5):451–9.

48. Bitter T, Langer C, Vogt J, et al. Sleep-disordered breathing in patients with atrial fibrillation and normal systolic left ventricular function. Dtsch Arztebl Int 2009;106(10):164–70.

49. Stevenson IH, Teichtahl H, Cunnington D, et al. Prevalence of sleep disordered breathing in paroxysmal and persistent atrial fibrillation patients with normal left ventricular function. Eur Heart J 2008; 29(13):1662–9.

50. Bazan V, Grau N, Valles E, et al. Obstructive sleep apnea in patients with typical atrial flutter: prevalence and impact on arrhythmia control outcome. Chest 2013;143(5):1277–83.

51. Abed HS, Wittert GA, Leong DP, et al. Effect of weight reduction and cardiometabolic risk factor management on symptom burden and severity in patients with atrial fibrillation: a randomized clinical trial. JAMA 2013;310(19):2050–60.

52. Grimm W, Becker HF. Obesity, sleep apnea syndrome, and rhythmogenic risk. Herz 2006;31(3): 213–8 [quiz: 219].

53. Pedrosa RP, Drager LF, Genta PR, et al. Obstructive sleep apnea is common and independently associated with atrial fibrillation in patients with hypertrophic cardiomyopathy. Chest 2010;137(5): 1078–84.

54. May AM, Blackwell T, Stone PH, et al. Central sleep-disordered breathing predicts incident atrial fibrillation in older men. Am J Respir Crit Care Med 2016;193(7):783–91.

55. Albuquerque FN, Kuniyoshi FH, Calvin AD, et al. Sleep-disordered breathing, hypertension, and

obesity in retired National Football League players. J Am Coll Cardiol 2010;56(17):1432–3.

56. Johns MW. A new method for measuring daytime sleepiness: the Epworth Sleepiness Scale. Sleep 1991;14(6):540–5.

57. Oldenburg O, Arzt M, Bitter T, et al. Positions papier "Schlafmedizin in der Kardiologie". Kardiologe 2015;9(2):140–58.

58. Szymanski FM, Filipiak KJ, Karpinski G, et al. Occurrence of poor sleep quality in atrial fibrillation patients according to the EHRA score. Acta Cardiol 2014;69(3):291–6.

59. Koshino Y, Villarraga HR, Orban M, et al. Changes in left and right ventricular mechanics during the Mueller maneuver in healthy adults: a possible mechanism for abnormal cardiac function in patients with obstructive sleep apnea. Circ Cardiovasc Imaging 2010;3(3):282–9.

60. Iwasaki YK, Kato T, Xiong F, et al. Atrial fibrillation promotion with long-term repetitive obstructive sleep apnea in a rat model. J Am Coll Cardiol 2014;64(19):2013–23.

61. Dimitri H, Ng M, Brooks AG, et al. Atrial remodeling in obstructive sleep apnea: implications for atrial fibrillation. Heart Rhythm 2012;9(3):321–7.

62. Iwasaki YK, Shi Y, Benito B, et al. Determinants of atrial fibrillation in an animal model of obesity and acute obstructive sleep apnea. Heart Rhythm 2012;9(9):1409–16.e1.

63. Altekin RE, Yanikoglu A, Karakas MS, et al. Assessment of left atrial dysfunction in obstructive sleep apnea patients with the two dimensional speckle-tracking echocardiography. Clin Res Cardiol 2012;101(6):403–13.

64. Shamsuzzaman AS, Winnicki M, Lanfranchi P, et al. Elevated C-reactive protein in patients with obstructive sleep apnea. Circulation 2002; 105(21):2462–4.

65. Schmalgemeier H, Bitter T, Fischbach T, et al. C-reactive protein is elevated in heart failure patients with central sleep apnea and Cheyne-Stokes respiration. Respiration 2014;87(2):113–20.

66. Monahan K, Brewster J, Wang L, et al. Relation of the severity of obstructive sleep apnea in response to anti-arrhythmic drugs in patients with atrial fibrillation or atrial flutter. Am J Cardiol 2012;110(3): 369–72.

67. Kanagala R, Murali NS, Friedman PA, et al. Obstructive sleep apnea and the recurrence of atrial fibrillation. Circulation 2003;107(20):2589–94.

68. Bitter T, Nolker G, Vogt J, et al. Predictors of recurrence in patients undergoing cryoballoon ablation for treatment of atrial fibrillation: the independent role of sleep-disordered breathing. J Cardiovasc Electrophysiol 2012;23(1):18–25.

69. Naruse Y, Tada H, Satoh M, et al. Concomitant obstructive sleep apnea increases the recurrence

of atrial fibrillation following radiofrequency catheter ablation of atrial fibrillation: clinical impact of continuous positive airway pressure therapy. Heart Rhythm 2013;10(3):331–7.

70. Fein AS, Shvilkin A, Shah D, et al. Treatment of obstructive sleep apnea reduces the risk of atrial fibrillation recurrence after catheter ablation. J Am Coll Cardiol 2013;62(4):300–5.

71. Walia HK, Chung MK, Ibrahim S, et al. Positive airway pressure-induced conversion of atrial fibrillation to normal sinus rhythm in severe obstructive sleep apnea. J Clin Sleep Med 2016;12(9):1301–3.

72. Patel D, Mohanty P, Di Biase L, et al. Safety and efficacy of pulmonary vein antral isolation in patients with obstructive sleep apnea: the impact of continuous positive airway pressure. Circ Arrhythm Electrophysiol 2010;3(5):445–51.

73. Arntz HR, Willich SN, Schreiber C, et al. Diurnal, weekly and seasonal variation of sudden death. Population-based analysis of 24,061 consecutive cases. Eur Heart J 2000;21(4):315–20.

74. Gami AS, Howard DE, Olson EJ, et al. Day-night pattern of sudden death in obstructive sleep apnea. N Engl J Med 2005;352(12):1206–14.

75. Gami AS, Olson EJ, Shen WK, et al. Obstructive sleep apnea and the risk of sudden cardiac death: a longitudinal study of 10,701 adults. J Am Coll Cardiol 2013;62(7):610–6.

76. Macedo PG, Brugada J, Leinveber P, et al. Sleep-disordered breathing in patients with the Brugada syndrome. Am J Cardiol 2011;107(5):709–13.

77. Grimm W, Apelt S, Timmesfeld N, et al. Sleep-disordered breathing in patients with implantable cardioverter-defibrillator. Europace 2013;15(4):515–22.

78. Prinz C, Bitter T, Oldenburg O, et al. Incidence of sleep-disordered breathing in patients with hypertrophic cardiomyopathy. Congest Heart Fail 2011; 17(1):19–24.

79. Fox H, Purucker HC, Holzhacker I, et al. Prevalence of sleep-disordered breathing and patient characteristics in a coronary artery disease cohort undergoing cardiovascular rehabilitation. J Cardiopulm Rehabil Prev 2016;36(6):421–9.

80. Bradley TD, Hall MJ, Ando S, et al. Hemodynamic effects of simulated obstructive apneas in humans with and without heart failure. Chest 2001;119(6): 1827–35.

81. Rossi VA, Stoewhas AC, Camen G, et al. The effects of continuous positive airway pressure therapy withdrawal on cardiac repolarization: data from a randomized controlled trial. Eur Heart J 2012;33(17):2206–12.

82. Barta K, Szabo Z, Kun C, et al. The effect of sleep apnea on QT interval, QT dispersion, and arrhythmias. Clin Cardiol 2010;33(6):E35–9.

83. Roche F, Gaspoz JM, Court-Fortune I, et al. Alteration of QT rate dependence reflects cardiac

autonomic imbalance in patients with obstructive sleep apnea syndrome. Pacing Clin Electrophysiol 2003;26(7 Pt 1):1446–53.

84. Takasugi N, Nishigaki K, Kubota T, et al. Sleep apnoea induces cardiac electrical instability assessed by T-wave alternans in patients with congestive heart failure. Eur J Heart Fail 2009; 11(11):1063–70.

85. Voigt L, Haq SA, Mitre CA, et al. Effect of obstructive sleep apnea on QT dispersion: a potential mechanism of sudden cardiac death. Cardiology 2011;118(1):68–73.

86. Shepard JW Jr, Garrison MW, Grither DA, et al. Relationship of ventricular ectopy to oxyhemoglobin desaturation in patients with obstructive sleep apnea. Chest 1985;88(3):335–40.

87. Bitter T, Westerheide N, Prinz C, et al. Cheyne-Stokes respiration and obstructive sleep apnoea are independent risk factors for malignant ventricular arrhythmias requiring appropriate cardioverter-defibrillator therapies in patients with congestive heart failure. Eur Heart J 2011;32(1):61–74.

88. Mehra R, Benjamin EJ, Shahar E, et al. Association of nocturnal arrhythmias with sleep-disordered breathing: the Sleep Heart Health study. Am J Respir Crit Care Med 2006;173(8):910–6.

89. Monahan K, Storfer-Isser A, Mehra R, et al. Triggering of nocturnal arrhythmias by sleep-disordered breathing events. J Am Coll Cardiol 2009;54(19):1797–804.

90. Bitter T, Gutleben KJ, Nolker G, et al. Treatment of Cheyne-Stokes respiration reduces arrhythmic events in chronic heart failure. J Cardiovasc Electrophysiol 2013;24(10):1132–40.

91. Cowie MR, Woehrle H, Wegscheider K, et al. Adaptive servo-ventilation for central sleep apnea in systolic heart failure. N Engl J Med 2015;373(12): 1095–105.

92. Lanfranchi PA, Somers VK, Braghiroli A, et al. Central sleep apnea in left ventricular dysfunction: prevalence and implications for arrhythmic risk. Circulation 2003;107(5):727–32.

93. Fichter J, Bauer D, Arampatzis S, et al. Sleep-related breathing disorders are associated with ventricular arrhythmias in patients with an implantable cardioverter-defibrillator. Chest 2002;122(2): 558–61.

94. Omran H, Bitter T, Fox H, et al. Association of sleep-disordered breathing and malignant arrhythmias in patients with ischemic and dilated cardiomyopathy. Herzschrittmacherther Elektrophysiol 2015;26(1):27–31 [in German].

95. Tomaello L, Zanolla L, Vassanelli C, et al. Sleep disordered breathing is associated with appropriate implantable cardioverter defibrillator therapy in congestive heart failure patients. Clin Cardiol 2010;33(2):E27–30.

96. Kreuz J, Skowasch D, Horlbeck F, et al. Usefulness of sleep-disordered breathing to predict occurrence of appropriate and inappropriate implantable-cardioverter defibrillator therapy in patients with implantable cardioverter-defibrillator for primary prevention of sudden cardiac death. Am J Cardiol 2013;111(9):1319–23.

97. Brignole M, Auricchio A, Baron-Esquivias G, et al. 2013 ESC Guidelines on cardiac pacing and cardiac resynchronization therapy: the Task Force on cardiac pacing and resynchronization therapy of the European Society of Cardiology (ESC). Developed in collaboration with the European Heart Rhythm Association (EHRA). Eur Heart J 2013; 34(29):2281–329.

98. Daubert JP, Zareba W, Cannom DS, et al. Inappropriate implantable cardioverter-defibrillator shocks in MADIT II: frequency, mechanisms, predictors, and survival impact. J Am Coll Cardiol 2008; 51(14):1357–65.

99. Bitter T, Gutleben KJ, Nolker G, et al. Sleep-disordered breathing and inappropriate defibrillator shocks in chronic heart failure. Herzschrittmacherther Elektrophysiol 2014;25(3):198–205.

100. Guilleminault C, Connolly SJ, Winkle RA. Cardiac arrhythmia and conduction disturbances during sleep in 400 patients with sleep apnea syndrome. Am J Cardiol 1983;52(5):490–4.

101. Koehler U, Fus E, Grimm W, et al. Heart block in patients with obstructive sleep apnoea: pathogenetic factors and effects of treatment. Eur Respir J 1998;11(2):434–9.

102. Miller WP. Cardiac arrhythmias and conduction disturbances in the sleep apnea syndrome. Prevalence and significance. Am J Med 1982;73(3): 317–21.

103. Becker H, Brandenburg U, Peter JH, et al. Reversal of sinus arrest and atrioventricular conduction block in patients with sleep apnea during nasal continuous positive airway pressure. Am J Respir Crit Care Med 1995;151(1):215–8.

104. Grimm W, Koehler U, Fus E, et al. Outcome of patients with sleep apnea-associated severe bradyarrhythmias after continuous positive airway pressure therapy. Am J Cardiol 2000;86(6):688–92. A689.

105. Simantirakis EN, Schiza SI, Marketou ME, et al. Severe bradyarrhythmias in patients with sleep apnoea: the effect of continuous positive airway pressure treatment: a long-term evaluation using an insertable loop recorder. Eur Heart J 2004; 25(12):1070–6.

106. Bitter T, Fox H, Dimitriadis Z, et al. Circadian variation of defibrillator shocks in patients with chronic heart failure: the impact of Cheyne-Stokes respiration and obstructive sleep apnea. Int J Cardiol 2014;176(3):1033–5.

107. Eulenburg C, Wegscheider K, Woehrle H, et al. Mechanisms underlying increased mortality risk in patients with heart failure and reduced ejection fraction randomly assigned to adaptive servoventilation in the SERVE-HF study: results of a secondary multistate modelling analysis. Lancet Respir Med 2016;4(11):873–81.

108. Javaheri S, Brown LK, Randerath W, et al. SERVE-hf: more questions than answers. Chest 2016; 149(4):900–4.

109. McEvoy RD, Antic NA, Heeley E, et al. CPAP for prevention of cardiovascular events in obstructive sleep apnea. N Engl J Med 2016;375(10):919–31.

110. Strollo PJ Jr, Soose RJ, Maurer JT, et al. Upper-airway stimulation for obstructive sleep apnea. N Engl J Med 2014;370(2):139–49.

111. Fox H, Bitter T, Gutleben KJ, et al. Cardiac or other implantable electronic devices and sleep-disordered breathing—implications for diagnosis and therapy. Arrhythm Electrophysiol Rev 2014; 3(2):116–9.

112. Fox H, Oldenburg O, Nolker G, et al. Detection and therapy of respiratory dysfunction by implantable (cardiac) devices. Herz 2014;39(1):32–6 [in German].

113. Costanzo MR, Ponikowski P, Javaheri S, et al. Transvenous neurostimulation for central sleep apnoea: a randomised controlled trial. Lancet 2016;388(10048):974–82.

114. Fiuzat M, Oldenberg O, Whellan DJ, et al. Lessons learned from a clinical trial: design, rationale, and insights from the cardiovascular improvements with Minute ventilation-targeted adaptive servo-ventilation (ASV) therapy in heart failure (CAT-HF) study. Contemp Clin Trials 2016;47:158–64.

115. Bitter T, Faber L, Hering D, et al. Sleep-disordered breathing in heart failure with normal left ventricular ejection fraction. Eur J Heart Fail 2009;11(6):602–8.

116. Bitter T, Westerheide N, Faber L, et al. Adaptive servoventilation in diastolic heart failure and Cheyne-Stokes respiration. Eur Respir J 2010; 36(2):385–92.

Device Therapy for Sleep-Disordered Breathing in Patients with Cardiovascular Diseases and Heart Failure

Winfried Randerath, MD*, Simon Herkenrath, MD

KEYWORDS

- Periodic breathing • Adaptive servoventilation • Loop gain • Bilevel spontaneous/timed mode

KEY POINTS

- Obstructive sleep apnea (OSA) is a key risk factors of arterial hypertension, atrial fibrillation, heart failure, and stroke.
- These cardiovascular diseases induce central sleep-related breathing disturbances, central sleep apnea (CSA), and periodic breathing.
- OSA and CSA are associated with poor outcome in patients with underlying cardiovascular diseases.
- PAP therapies improve sleepiness, quality of life, cardiac function, and outcome in patients with symptomatic OSA and cardiovascular diseases.
- Outcomes in chronic systolic heart failure and CSA treated with PAP therapy are debated.

RELEVANCE OF BREATHING DISTURBANCES DURING SLEEP IN CARDIOVASCULAR PATIENTS

Cardiovascular diseases and sleep-related breathing disturbances (SRDB) are associated in a bidirectional relationship. On the one hand, obstructive sleep apnea (OSA) has been acknowledged as an independent risk factor for arterial hypertension, atrial fibrillation, chronic systolic heart failure, and cerebrovascular diseases. The characteristic change between hypoxia and reoxygenation and the catecholamine release owing to arousals from sleep are associated with systemic inflammation, oxidative stress, hypoxia of the adipocytes, and metabolic alterations, including insulin resistance of the skeletal muscle, release of free fatty acids, and fat deposition in the liver. Thus, OSA is associated with atherosclerosis, vascular thrombosis, left ventricular hypertrophy, and adverse cardiac remodeling.[1]

In contrast, heart failure with reduced ejection fraction or preserved left ventricular ejection fraction frequently induces central SRDB. They are characterized by chronic hyperventilation and increased peripheral and central chemosensitivity. As a consequence, ventilation is upregulated and the respiratory loop gain is elevated, which induces a continuous shift between overshooting and undershooting of the ventilation. Patients present with the polysomnographic phenotypes of periodic breathing (PB), that is, a switch between the extremes of hyperventilation and hypoventilation or central sleep apnea (CSA; **Fig. 1**).[2]

Financial Disclosure: Dr W. Randerath reports grants and personal fees from Inspire, Resmed, Philips Respironics, Weinmann and Heinen & Löwenstein outside the submitted work.
Clinic for Pneumology and Allergology, Centre of Sleep Medicine and Respiratory Care, Bethanien Hospital, Institute of Pneumology, University of Cologne, Aufderhöher Str. 169, Solingen 42699, Germany
* Corresponding author.
E-mail address: randerath@klinik-bethanien.de

Sleep Med Clin 12 (2017) 243–254
http://dx.doi.org/10.1016/j.jsmc.2017.02.002
1556-407X/17/© 2017 Elsevier Inc. All rights reserved.

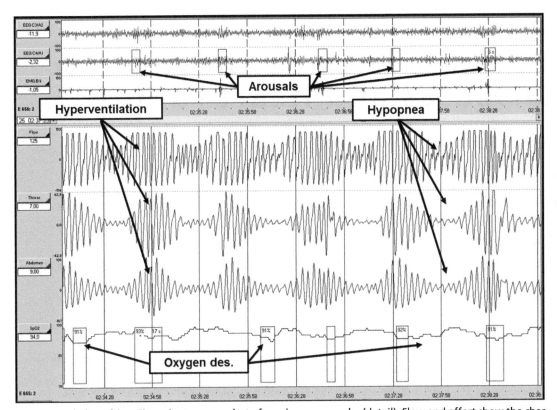

Fig. 1. Periodic breathing. Five-minute screen shot of a polysomnography (detail). Flow and effort show the characteristic waxing and waning pattern (crescendo–decrescendo) of periodic breathing. The ventilation varies between hyperventilation and hypoventilation. The periods of hyperventilation are followed by hypopneas—not apneas—in this example. Arousals appear at the maximum of ventilation, which is typical of periodic breathing. Channels from top to bottom: 2 electroencephalography channels, electromyography, flow (pressure transducer at the nose), thoracic and abdominal effort belts, oxygen saturation (finger plethysmography, SpO₂). des., desaturation.

SRDB in cardiovascular disorders are of crucial relevance owing to their prevalence and the impact on patient outcomes. Several studies have shown that at least 50% of heart failure patients present with SRBD, almost equally divided in OSA and CSA/PB.[3] Patients with heart failure and SRBD differ substantially from those without CSA. Khayat and colleagues[4] most recently showed that survival of patients hospitalized for acute cardiac failure with OSA or CSA was significantly reduced over a follow-up of 36 months. Exercise performance and quality of life are reduced in heart failure patients with PB.[5,6] Severe HCSB predisposes to arrhythmias, likely owing to increased sympathetic activity.[7,8] In a recent review, Brack and colleagues[3] summarized data from cohorts, longitudinal studies, and retrospective analyses addressing the impact of CSA in patients with severe heart failure with reduced ejection fraction (left ventricular ejection fraction [LVEF] of 20%–36%). The risk of death was

independently increased in heart failure patients with PB (HR 2.1–5.7 in 5 of 7 studies).[3] However, many of the heart failure patients with CSA/PB do not present with the classical symptoms of sleep apnea.[9] Therefore, a systematic screening for SRBD in patients with cardiovascular diseases seems to be reasonable.[10]

THE HETEROGENEITY OF THE PHENOTYPES OF SLEEP-RELATED BREATHING DISTURBANCES

In clinical practice, the majority of patients do not suffer from pure obstructive or central SRBD, but from combinations of both in various portions. Nevertheless, most studies arbitrarily classify the phenotypes of OSA and CSA by the majority of apneas, that is, a patient's disease is diagnosed as OSA if more than 50% of the apneas fulfill the obstructive criteria (**Fig. 2**). In addition, many investigators abstain from any differentiation of

Predominant phenotype?

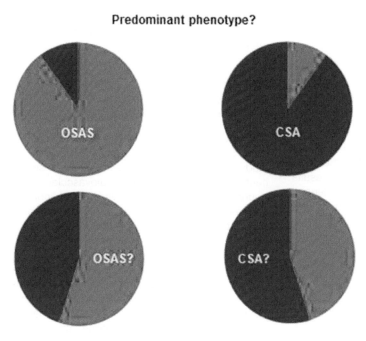

Fig. 2. Differentiation of obstructive and central phenotypes. The figures demonstrate schematically the difficulty of defining a precise diagnosis of the phenotypes of sleep-related breathing disturbances. The colors show the relative amounts of obstructive and central apneas in different polysomnographies. Both left-side circles present patients with predominant obstructive sleep apnea syndrome (OSAS), the right-side circles predominant central sleep apnea (CSA). Obviously, these labels fit well to the upper examples. However, the simplified diagnoses clearly underestimate the relevance of the minor component in the lower examples.

hypopneas, although they often represent the majority of SRDB. These simplifications of the heterogeneity of the clinical situations may impede interpretation of scientific studies and sufficient treatment. To select the optimal treatment option, a precise differentiation of the events and description of the disease seems to be crucial.[11]

OBSTRUCTIVE SLEEP APNEA: FUNCTIONAL AND MECHANICAL ASPECTS

The diameter of the upper airways depends on the relation between the intraluminal and extraluminal pressures, the pressure within the airways, and the surrounding tissue. The extraluminal pressure may exceed the intraluminal pressure in obesity or craniofacial malformations, and thus predisposes to partial (hypopnea) or complete (apnea) closing of the upper airways. The effect is intensified in cardiovascular patients owing to a fluid shift from the lower to the upper body compartments in the supine position.[12] However, dilating muscles of the upper airways counterbalance the collapsing forces during wakefulness; however, this compensation often fails during sleep, especially REM sleep.[13] The mechanical effects can be quantified by the critical closing pressure, which is defined by the level of the intraluminal pressure below which the upper airway collapses.[14] In addition to the morphologic components and failure of the muscular compensation, obstructions of the upper

airways are also associated with increased respiratory drive.[15]

POSITIVE AIRWAY PRESSURE THERAPY IN OBSTRUCTIVE SLEEP APNEA

Because intensive education of patients on sleep behavior and weight reduction are often insufficient as a single measures,[16] additional treatment options are required, particularly in patients with coexisting cardiovascular disease. The application of positive airway pressures (PAP) has proven effective to increase intraluminal pressure and overcome upper airway obstruction. It is provided by a flow generator device and applied to the patient via a tube and a facial or orofacial mask. In contrast with alternative treatment options, such as mandibular advancement devices, PAP stabilizes the upper airways independent of the localization of the obstruction.[17]

PAP devices use different algorithms:

- Continuous PAP (CPAP).
- Automatically varying pressures according to the actual level of obstruction (automatic PAP [APAP]).
- Two different, but fixed inspiratory and expiratory pressure levels (bilevel airway pressure [BPAP]).

These algorithms are equally sufficient in suppressing obstructive events.[18–20] They improve sleep quality, daytime performance, and neurocognitive deficits, and reduce motor vehicle accidents.

EFFECTS OF CONTINUOUS POSITIVE AIRWAY PRESSURE IN PATIENTS WITH CARDIOVASCULAR DISORDERS AND OBSTRUCTIVE SLEEP APNEA

Several studies have addressed the influence of CPAP on cardiovascular comorbidities in patients with OSAS. The general effect of PAP therapies on arterial hypertension is limited, but the results of the available investigations may be influenced by the inclusion of nonhypertensive or pharmaceutically well-treated patients and by nonadherence to CPAP therapy. However, Kohler and colleagues[21] found significant reductions in the vascular augmentation index and the mean arterial blood pressure in effectively treated patients. In addition, CPAP has been shown to improve blood pressure in patients with treatment-refractory hypertension and CPAP-adherent patients. Campos-Rodriguez and associates[22] found a significant improvement after 24 months of CPAP in patients with insufficiently controlled hypertension and in those who used their devices for more than 3.5 hours per day. Baseline systolic blood pressure and hourly use of CPAP were independent predictors of improvements under CPAP. Similarly, in a randomized, controlled trial showed that CPAP significantly decreased blood pressure in moderate to severe hypertension by about 10 mm Hg.[23]

Although only limited data are available, the beneficial effects of optimally applied CPAP have also been shown in coronary artery disease.[24] Peker and colleagues[25] presented the data of a prospective, randomized, controlled trial in nonsleepy OSA patients. After cardiac revascularization therapy, the patients were randomized to receive CPAP in addition to conventional cardiac therapy or standard care alone. After a mean follow-up of 57 months, there was no difference in the primary combined cardiovascular endpoint. However, adjusted on-treatment analysis showed a significant risk reduction in those who used CPAP for 4 or more hours per day as compared with insufficient users or those who did not receive treatment (hazard ratio, 0.29; 95% confidence interval, 0.10–0.86; $P = .026$).

Qureshi and colleagues[26] performed a systematic review on the efficacy of CPAP on atrial fibrillation. They analyzed data from 698 CPAP users and 549 nonusers in 8 studies. The risk of atrial fibrillation in sufficiently treated patients was 0.58 in sufficiently treated patients (95% confidence interval, 0.47–0.70). In metaregression analysis, the benefits of CPAP were stronger for younger, obese, and male patients ($P<.05$). Moreover, CPAP therapy and atrial fibrillation recurrence were correlated inversely.

PROGNOSTIC IMPACT OF CONTINUOUS POSITIVE AIRWAY PRESSURE IN OBSTRUCTIVE SLEEP APNEA

The prognostic impact of PAP in patients with OSA is under debate.[27–29] In a large, observational study, Marin and colleagues[30] showed significantly more life-threatening cardiovascular events in untreated patients with severe OSA syndrome apnea–hypopnea index ([AHI] ≥30/h) as compared with untreated patients with lesser degrees of the disease, simple snorers, healthy controls, and patients treated effectively with CPAP. Similarly, Buchner and colleagues[24] compared the outcome of 364 effectively treated and adherent patients and 85 patients who refused treatment after 72 months follow-up. Effective CPAP therapy was associated with a substantial reduction in fatal and nonfatal cardiovascular events. Most recently, McEvoy and colleagues[28] investigated the influence of CPAP in addition to usual care as compared with usual care alone in patients with moderate to severe OSA and a history of cardiovascular diseases (SAVE trial [CPAP for prevention of cardiovascular events in obstructive sleep apnea]). A vast majority of the patients were under treatment with antihypertensive and antithrombotic agents, indicating optimal medical treatment. The study failed to show a difference in the primary composite cardiovascular endpoint (death from cardiovascular causes, myocardial infarction, stroke, and hospitalization for unstable angina, heart failure, or transient ischemic attack). However, CPAP significantly improved quality of life, daytime sleepiness, anxiety, and depression as measured by validated questionnaires. Moreover, the numbers of accidents causing injury and the days off from work because of poor health were substantially reduced with CPAP. There was a clear trend ($P = .05$) toward reduction of strokes and a significant reduction of combined cerebral events in those patients who were CPAP adherent. The results of the SAVE trial have to be discussed cautiously.

- The mean daily use of CPAP was only 3.3 h/d, which is clearly below the recommendations for sufficient compliance. Although the SAVE patients suffered from moderate to severe sleep apnea as measured by the AHI, the sleepiness score was in the normal range. The mild symptoms may have influenced CPAP usage.[31]

- CPAP was applied in patients with predetermined manifest cardiovascular diseases under optimal conventional treatment (secondary prevention). Obviously, the room for improvement for a treatment focusing on a risk factor is quite limited.

Although CPAP cannot generally be recommended in patients with optimally treated cardiovascular diseases without daytime symptoms based on the SAVE results, the data clearly support treatment for those patients who suffer from daytime sleepiness or impaired quality of life. The study does not allow any conclusions on the efficacy of CPAP in the primary prevention of cardiovascular outcome.

CONTINUOUS POSITIVE AIRWAY PRESSURE THERAPY IN HEART FAILURE AND PREDOMINANT OBSTRUCTIVE SLEEP APNEA

In patients with OSA and heart failure, CPAP has additional effects on oxygenation and cardiac function[32–39] (**Table 1**). As a consequence, several—although not all—randomized, controlled trials have shown increases of the LVEF.[40–42] Moreover, Javaheri and colleagues[43] showed a significant improvement in survival of those patients diagnosed and treated for sleep apnea in a large, population-based, observational study in patients with newly diagnosed heart failure. A significant survival benefit was confirmed in a small observational study[44] in CPAP-adherent heart failure patients with OSA.

PATHOPHYSIOLOGY OF CENTRAL BREATHING DISTURBANCES DURING SLEEP

Besides upper airway obstruction, sufficient ventilation depends on respiratory drive and tidal volume. Minute ventilation correlates linearly with the level of carbon dioxide (CO_2) in blood and cerebrospinal fluid. Hypoventilation (characterized by hypercapnia, increased level of CO_2) stimulates ventilatory drive, increases breathing frequency and—if possible—tidal volume. In contrast, hypocapnia (reduction of CO_2) dampens respiration.

The term "loop gain" is often used to quantify the ratio of ventilatory response to a disturbance in ventilation.[45] Respiratory drive may be decreased, that is, the loop gain of ventilation is reduced, leading to hypercapnic failure with or without central apneas. Patients with heart failure often present with an increased loop gain. The response of the ventilatory system is upregulated, as characterized by the overshoot of ventilation to hypercapnia and hypoxia and by the undershoot in response to hypocapnia. The system is unstable; patients clinically and polysomnographically present with a PB pattern, including hypocapnic central apneas (nonhypercapnic CSA).[2,46,47] Increased chemosensitivity, reduced lung volume owing to the fluid accumulation, stimulation of intrapulmonary vagal afferents, and increased circulation time but also frequent arousals from sleep contribute to the increased loop gain in heart failure patients.[48–50] Sympathetic activity, malignant cardiac arrhythmias, and mortality are increased in heart failure patients with CSA as compared with those without breathing disturbances.[32,51–56]

CONTINUOUS POSITIVE AIRWAY PRESSURE IN THE TREATMENT OF CENTRAL BREATHING DISTURBANCES

Before PAP treatment of central SRBD, optimal interventional and pharmaceutical therapy of any underlying disorder should be reevaluated critically.[57,58] However, if a patient suffers from symptoms related to poor quality of sleep or cardiac impairment not responding to standard therapies, specific treatment of SRBD may be justified. As pointed out, the application of CPAP may influence cardiac function substantially owing to improved oxygenation and mechanical factors. Although improvements of the LVEF have been confirmed repeatedly, this did not translate in

Table 1		
Effects of continuous positive airway pressure on heart function		
Mechanism	**Effect**	
Reduction the high intrathoracic pressure swings	Reduction of work of breathing Reduction of oxygen demand	
Shifting of interstitial fluid into the vascular bed	Improvement of ventilation–perfusion mismatches Improvement of oxygenation	
Elimination of apneas and hypopneas	Reduction of work of breathing Improvement of oxygenation	
Reduction of left ventricular afterload	Improvement of cardiac output	
Reduction of stimulation of intrapulmonary vagal afferents	Dampening of ventilatory overshoot	

increased survival rates in large, prospective, randomized studies so far.[44,59] Although the Canadian Continuous Positive Airway Pressure (CanPAP) trial showed that CPAP improved apneas and hypopneas, oxygen saturation, ejection fraction, norepinephrine levels, and exercise performance over a mean of 2 years, it failed to prove a survival benefit.[59] Interestingly, a non-predefined post hoc analysis found a significantly better outcome in CPAP responders as compared with nonresponders. These data have to be discussed cautiously because CPAP response might on the one hand indicate an impact of treatment on survival or on the other hand select a specific, prognostically better phenotype.[60]

The heterogeneity of the treatment response has been elucidated by Sands and colleagues.[61] These investigators calculated the loop gain in animal trials and heart failure patients and found a high loop gain, that is, a highly unstable respiratory system, to be associated with poor response to PAP therapy. In contrast, a dampened loop gain showed better treatment response. The implementation of these findings into clinical practice might allow physicians to predict possible PAP effects before treatment and individually select therapeutic options.

However, for today, CPAP is the first step in the treatment of central breathing disturbances refractory to conventional therapy of the underlying diseases. As compared with more sophisticated devices such as adaptive servoventilation (ASV), CPAP is simple, cheap, and commonly available. In contrast with OSA, APAP or BPAP cannot replace CPAP in patients with CSA with increased loop gain:

- There is no sufficient scientific evidence to recommend APAP or BPAP in patients with PB or nonhypercapnic CSA.
- Serious concerns rise from pathophysiologic considerations: CPAP does not only influence upper airway diameters but also lung volumes (functional residual capacity) and ventilation–perfusion mismatches. APAP devices apply the lowest possible pressure to overcome upper airway obstruction, resulting in a reduction of mean pressures as compared with CPAP. This may miss the pressure level required to improve parameters of lung function or oxygenation.
- BPAP devices apply 2 different pressure levels during inspiration (IPAP) and expiration (EPAP). The change between IPAP and EPAP is achieved by a volume shift. In addition, BPAP can be used with or without application of mandatory breaths (timed mode or

spontaneous mode, respectively). This mechanical ventilation may further reduce carbon dioxide, enhance the high loop gain and the ventilatory instability in patients with nonhypercapnic CSA (including heart failure).

ADAPTIVE SERVOVENTILATION

ASV is a modification of BPAP, which variably addresses the pathologic changes of the PB pattern. It increases the pressure difference between inspiration and expiration (the tidal volume) during hypoventilation and decreases it during hyperventilation. Devices from different manufacturers and different generations of ASV algorithms differ in target parameters, sensing of the ventilatory parameters, and pattern of reaction.[62,63]

EVOLUTION OF ADAPTIVE SERVOVENTILATION ALGORITHMS

The first versions of the algorithms applied a minimal pressure support of 3 mbar even in periods of hyperventilation—an aspect that might be relevant for further discussions (see below). In contrast, the most recent releases of the devices reduce the IPAP to the expiratory level ("0" difference) and work in CPAP mode if no pressure support is required. To overcome any concomitant upper airway obstruction, the physician had to set the EPAP in the first ASV devices manually, often based on a previous CPAP titration. However, the actual algorithms measure flow limitations and automatically vary the EPAP level similar to APAP algorithms. In addition, some ASV devices vary the pressure between early and end-expiration. The airways are widest during the first part of expiration, allowing to reduce the early EPAP. However, to stabilize the airways, pressure is increased at the end of expiration (**Fig. 3**). Finally, the machines apply mandatory breaths to eliminate apneic events (**Box 1**).[62,63]

ADAPTIVE SERVOVENTILATION IN CHRONIC HEART FAILURE

ASV has proven to overcome obstructive components equally effectively as CPAP and to normalize ventilation in different subgroups of central breathing disturbances superior to all other therapeutic options (O_2, CPAP, BPAP-ST).[64–70] In congestive heart failure (CHF) patients, ASV reduces the hypercapnic ventilatory response—a key factor of nonhypercapnic CSA—and has been shown to be superior to CPAP in suppressing preexisting CSA and coexisting OSA and CSA.[64,67,68,71–76] Consecutively, recent data showed beneficial influences of ASV on quality of sleep in CHF with

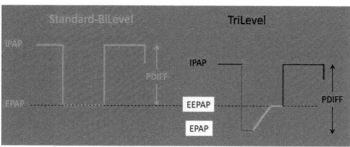

Fig. 3. Different pressure levels of ventilatory support. The difference between the inspiratory (IPAP) and the expiratory pressure level (EPAP) defines the tidal volume. Increases of the tidal volume may be required to overcome hypoventilation; EPAP stabilizes the upper airways to overcome obstructions. Some devices allow to reduce the EPAP during early expiration (EEPAP), the period of minimal obstruction throughout the breathing cycle. This leads to a reduction of the maximum pressure levels without change in the tidal volume. PDIFF, pressure difference.

central or OSA. Hetzenecker and colleagues[77] randomized 63 CHF patients to receive ASV or conventional cardiac treatment for 12 weeks. ASV reduced the total arousal index and the sleep fragmentation index, and improved sleep efficiency as compared with controls significantly. In addition, the same group analyzed retrospectively the effect of CPAP and ASV on parameters of respiration and sleep in 82 patients with severe CHF (LVEF 35% ± 16%). After a CPAP trial for 47 days, CPAP nonresponders were switched to ASV and responders continued using CPAP. As compared with the CPAP responders, ASV significantly reduced AHI, arousal index and improved REM sleep.[78]

Several studies have investigated the effect of ASV on cardiac function.[67,71,72,74,76] The algorithm sufficiently improved LVEF in systolic heart failure and cardiac surrogate parameters. Most recently, Toyama and colleagues[79] randomized 31 patients with heart failure with reduced ejection fraction and CSA to receive ASV or conventional treatment

for 6 months These investigators found significantly better improvement not only in AHI but also in LVEF, New York Heart Association functional class, and in the nuclear I-metaiodobenzylguanidine imaging. They concluded that improving cheyne stokes respiration (CSR)/CSA reduces sympathetic nerve activity and is therefore a factor of better outcome.

CONTROVERSIES ON THE PROGNOSTIC IMPACT OF ADAPTIVE SERVOVENTILATION

Takama and Kurabayashi[80] compared fatal cardiac events in 2 groups of CHF patients with New York Heart Association functional class II through IV under optimal conventional therapy with or without good adherence with ASV. They found an improvement of the 1-year survival rate in the ASV-treated patients using their devices for more than 4 hours per night (hazard ratio, 0.53; 95% confidence interval; 0.27–0.99). However, Cowie and colleagues[29] published the first large, multinational, prospective, randomized, controlled trial (SERVE-HF [Treatment of Predominant Central Sleep Apnea by Adaptive Servo Ventilation in Patients With Heart Failure]) on the effects of ASV as compared with standard care in patients with severe systolic CHF (LVEF <45%) and CSA. Although the primary combined cardiovascular endpoint did not differ significantly between the 2 groups, further analyses showed increased rates of death from any cause and cardiovascular death in the ASV group. In contrast with previous findings, the study failed to demonstrate beneficial effects on cardiac or quality of life parameters. Eulenburg and colleagues[81] performed a modeling analysis of the SERVE-HF data, asking for individual components influencing mortality. They showed an increased risk of cardiovascular death without previous hospital admission and cardiovascular death after a

---

Box 1
Characteristics of adaptive servoventilation devices

- IPAP: inspiratory positive airway pressure.
- EPAP: expiratory positive airway pressure at the end of expiration.
- EEPAP: early EPAP (not available in all devices).
- Difference between IPAP and EEPAP (if not available, EPAP), defining the pressure support and tidal volume.
- Mandatory breaths to overcome central apneas, independent if hypercapnic or hypocapnic.

life-saving event. These data suggest that not acute cardiac decompensation, but sudden cardiac death was responsible for the excess mortality. Moreover, they confirmed the subanalysis of the main paper showing that the increased mortality was limited to those patients with an LVEF of 30% or less.

OPEN QUESTIONS ON THE TREATMENT OF SLEEP-DISORDERED BREATHING WITH PREDOMINANT CENTRAL SLEEP APNEA BY ADAPTIVE SERVO VENTILATION IN PATIENTS WITH HEART FAILURE TRIAL

However, the methodology, analysis, and interpretation of the study raise several concerns.[47,82] The high cross-over between the treatment arms (23%) and the low compliance (27% of the patients <1 hour per night, 40% <3 hours per night) limit the conclusions of the study substantially. However, these limitations were not taken into account in the published analyses so far.[29,81] The intention-to-treat analysis does not reflect the real influence of ASV because it includes a huge portion of participants who were not or not sufficiently treated with the device. On the other hand, on-treatment analysis might be misleading owing to selection of generally highly compliant patients (also with all other therapies). Data on LVEF were missing in 19% of the patients,[81] although the inclusion criteria asked for an LVEF of less than 45%. The diagnosis was often based on polygraphy, not on polysomnography. However, polysomnography does not allow excluding central breathing disturbances in sleep–wake transitions or wakefulness, or differentiating of central and obstructive hypopneas according to arousal position and sleep stages.[11] These aspects might have led to the misclassification of respiratory disturbances, which may have influenced the inclusion of the patients.

Patients were treated with an old ASV version with fixed expiratory pressure and a minimal pressure support of 3 cm H_2O. This might have caused unnecessary ventilation owing to the unavoidable pressure support in periods of hyperventilation and to inadequately high fixed EPAP levels. It has been hypothesized that these factors may be associated with hypocapnia, electrolyte imbalance, and consecutive instability of cardiac cells.[82] Similarly, the unbalanced antiarrhythmic therapy might have contributed to destabilize cardiac rhythm and induce fatal events or may be a marker of more sensitive heart failure phenotypes. These considerations are supported by subanalyses showing higher mortality rates only in those patients using antiarrhythmic drugs and those with an LVEF of less than 30%.

The SERVE-HF investigators discussed the idea that PB may be a compensatory mechanism of the failing heart and, thus, the suppression of PB could be deleterious.[29] However, the facts that patients did not die from cardiac decompensation but from sudden cardiac death and that PAP therapy has been shown to improve cardiac output, sympathetic activity, and oxygenation disprove this idea.[33–39,83–85] Because the interpretation of SERVE-HF remains unclear so far, further analyses of the study are urgently required. Importantly, any subsequent analysis has to include the limitations of compliance and cross-over cautiously.

Contradictory data on survival have been published before and after SERVE-HF. Most recently, Khayat and colleagues[4] applied ASV to heart failure with reduced ejection fraction patients with newly diagnosed CSA who survived for 3 months after hospitalization for decompensated heart failure. Of 307 patients, 194 did not pursue any treatment for their CSA; 47 were treated with ASV and 66 with CPAP. After a median follow-up of 65 months, the hazard ratio for mortality after adjusting for age, sex, body mass index, AHI, LVEF, creatinine, atrial fibrillation, hypertension, coronary disease, chronic kidney disease, diabetes, and implantable cardioverter defibrillator status was 0.32 (95% confidence interval, 0.12–0.84; $P = .02$) in the ASV group versus the untreated group. In contrast with SERVE-HF, these data showed a protective effect of ASV. The results of the second, large-scale ASV trial (ADVENT-HF [Effect of Adaptive Servo Ventilation (ASV) on Survival and Hospital Admissions in Heart Failure]) are awaited because an interim analysis of the safety data supported continuing the study. Owing to a lack of survival data, oxygen, BPAP in spontaneous or timed mode, and phrenic nerve stimulation should also be used only in clinical trials for patients with severe heart failure with reduced ejection fraction.[57]

SUMMARY

The high prevalence and the poor outcome of obstructive and central breathing disturbances during sleep urge clinicians to thoroughly consider optimal therapy for patients with underlying cardiac diseases. PAP therapies stabilize the upper airways and improve oxygenation and cardiac mechanics. CPAP is the treatment of choice for patients with cardiovascular diseases and OSA. However, because it has not proven to improve outcome in secondary prevention in cardiac patients without daytime sleepiness, it should be recommended for symptomatic OSA patients. ASV improves respiratory disturbances, LVEF, quality of life, and sleep parameters in patients with chronic heart failure and CSA and PB. Symptomatic heart failure patients with predominant OSA and patients with CSA and preserved LVEF can undergo a trial of CPAP or, if it fails, ASV. However, based on the results of the SERVE-HF trial, for now ASV should not be used in CHF patients with severely impaired LVEF. Owing to pathophysiologic considerations or missing data, neither oxygen nor BPAP or other modalities can be recommended for this high-risk group. The limitations of SERVE-HF underline the necessity of further trials in these patients.

REFERENCES

1. Bonsignore MR, Esquinas C, Barcelo A, et al. Metabolic syndrome, insulin resistance and sleepiness in real-life obstructive sleep apnoea. Eur Respir J 2012;39(5):1136–43.
2. Randerath W, Javaheri S. Sleep-disordered breathing in patients with heart failure. Curr Sleep Med Rep 2016;2(2):99–106.
3. Brack T, Randerath W, Bloch KE. Cheyne-stokes respiration in patients with heart failure: prevalence, causes, consequences and treatments. Respiration 2012;83(2):165–76.
4. Khayat R, Jarjoura D, Porter K, et al. Sleep disordered breathing and post-discharge mortality in patients with acute heart failure. Eur Heart J 2015; 36(23):1463–9.
5. Walsh JT, Andrews R, Evans A, et al. Failure of "effective" treatment for heart failure to improve normal customary activity. Br Heart J 1995;74(4): 373–6.
6. Carmona-Bernal C, Ruiz-Garcia A, Villa-Gil M, et al. Quality of life in patients with congestive heart failure and central sleep apnea. Sleep Med 2008;9(6):646–51.
7. Lanfranchi PA, Somers VK, Braghiroli A, et al. Central sleep apnea in left ventricular dysfunction: prevalence and implications for arrhythmic risk. Circulation 2003;107(5):727–32.
8. Leung RS, Diep TM, Bowman ME, et al. Provocation of ventricular ectopy by Cheyne-Stokes respiration in patients with heart failure. Sleep 2004;27(7): 1337–43.
9. Arzt M, Young T, Finn L, et al. Sleepiness and sleep in patients with both systolic heart failure and obstructive sleep apnea. Arch Intern Med 2006; 166(16):1716–22.
10. Randerath W. Time for screening? Sleep Med 2014; 15(11):1285–6.
11. Randerath WJ, Treml M, Priegnitz C, et al. Evaluation of a noninvasive algorithm for differentiation of obstructive and central hypopneas. Sleep 2013; 36(3):363–8.
12. Yumino D, Redolfi S, Ruttanaumpawan P, et al. Nocturnal rostral fluid shift: a unifying concept for the pathogenesis of obstructive and central sleep apnea in men with heart failure. Circulation 2010; 121(14):1598–605.
13. McGinley BM, Schwartz AR, Schneider H, et al. Upper airway neuromuscular compensation during sleep is defective in obstructive sleep apnea. J Appl Physiol (1985) 2008;105(1):197–205.
14. Schwartz AR, Smith PL, Wise RA, et al. Induction of upper airway occlusion in sleeping individuals with subatmospheric nasal pressure. J Appl Physiol (1985) 1988;64(2):535–42.
15. Wellman A, Eckert DJ, Jordan AS, et al. A method for measuring and modeling the physiological traits causing obstructive sleep apnea. J Appl Physiol (1985) 2011;110(6):1627–37.
16. Randerath WJ, Verbraecken J, Andreas S, et al. Non-CPAP therapies in obstructive sleep apnea. Eur Respir J 2011;37(5):1000–28.
17. Sullivan CE, Issa FG, Berthon-Jones M, et al. Reversal of obstructive sleep apnoea by continuous positive airway pressure applied through the nares. Lancet 1981;1(8225):862–5.
18. Morgenthaler TI, Aurora RN, Brown T, et al. Practice parameters for the use of autotitrating continuous positive airway pressure devices for titrating pressures and treating adult patients with obstructive sleep apnea syndrome: an update for 2007. An American Academy of Sleep Medicine report. Sleep 2008;31(1):141–7.
19. Randerath WJ, Schraeder O, Galetke W, et al. Autoadjusting CPAP therapy based on impedance efficacy, compliance and acceptance. Am J Respir Crit Care Med 2001;163(3 Pt 1):652–7.
20. Randerath WJ, Galetke W, Ruhle KH. Auto-adjusting CPAP based on impedance versus bilevel pressure in difficult-to-treat sleep apnea syndrome: a prospective randomized crossover study. Med Sci Monit 2003;9(8):CR353–8.
21. Kohler M, Pepperell JC, Casadei B, et al. CPAP and measures of cardiovascular risk in males with OSAS. Eur Respir J 2008;32(6):1488–96.
22. Campos-Rodriguez F, Perez-Ronchel J, Grilo-Reina A, et al. Long-term effect of continuous positive airway pressure on BP in patients with hypertension and sleep apnea. Chest 2007;132(6): 1847–52.
23. Kaneko Y, Floras JS, Usui K, et al. Cardiovascular effects of continuous positive airway pressure in patients with heart failure and obstructive sleep apnea. N Engl J Med 2003;348(13):1233–41.
24. Buchner NJ, Sanner BM, Borgel J, et al. Continuous positive airway pressure treatment of mild to moderate obstructive sleep apnea reduces cardiovascular risk. Am J Respir Crit Care Med 2007; 176(12):1274–80.

25. Peker Y, Glantz H, Eulenburg C, et al. Effect of positive airway pressure on cardiovascular outcomes in coronary artery disease patients with nonsleepy obstructive sleep apnea. The RICCADSA randomized controlled trial. Am J Respir Crit Care Med 2016;194(5):613–20.

26. Qureshi WT, Nasir UB, Alqalyoobi S, et al. Meta-analysis of continuous positive airway pressure as a therapy of atrial fibrillation in obstructive sleep apnea. Am J Cardiol 2015;116(11):1767–73.

27. Bradley TD, Logan AG, Floras JS, et al. Rationale and design of the Canadian Continuous Positive Airway Pressure Trial for congestive heart failure patients with central sleep apnea–CANPAP. Can J Cardiol 2001;17(6):677–84.

28. McEvoy RD, Antic NA, Heeley E, et al. CPAP for prevention of cardiovascular events in obstructive sleep apnea. N Engl J Med 2016;375(10):919–31.

29. Cowie MR, Woehrle H, Wegscheider K, et al. Adaptive servo-ventilation for central sleep apnea in systolic heart failure. N Engl J Med 2015;373(12):1095–105.

30. Marin JM, Carrizo SJ, Vicente E, et al. Long-term cardiovascular outcomes in men with obstructive sleep apnoea-hypopnoea with or without treatment with continuous positive airway pressure: an observational study. Lancet 2005;365(9464):1046–53.

31. Weaver TE, Maislin G, Dinges DF, et al. Relationship between hours of CPAP use and achieving normal levels of sleepiness and daily functioning. Sleep 2007;30(6):711–9.

32. Javaheri S. Effects of continuous positive airway pressure on sleep apnea and ventricular irritability in patients with heart failure. Circulation 2000;101(4):392–7.

33. Tobin MJ. Mechanical ventilation. N Engl J Med 1994;330(15):1056–61.

34. Smith TC, Marini JJ. Impact of PEEP on lung mechanics and work of breathing in severe airflow obstruction. J Appl Physiol (1985) 1988;65(4):1488–99.

35. Esteban A, Anzueto A, Frutos F, et al. Characteristics and outcomes in adult patients receiving mechanical ventilation: a 28-day international study. JAMA 2002;287(3):345–55.

36. de Miguel J, Cabello J, Sanchez-Alarcos JM, et al. Long-term effects of treatment with nasal continuous positive airway pressure on lung function in patients with overlap syndrome. Sleep Breath 2002;6(1):3–10.

37. Petrof BJ, Legare M, Goldberg P, et al. Continuous positive airway pressure reduces work of breathing and dyspnea during weaning from mechanical ventilation in severe chronic obstructive pulmonary disease. Am Rev Respir Dis 1990;141(2):281–9.

38. Verbraecken J, Willemen M, De Cock W, et al. Continuous positive airway pressure and lung inflation in sleep apnea patients. Respiration 2001;68(4):357–64.

39. Malo J, Ali J, Wood LD. How does positive end-expiratory pressure reduce intrapulmonary shunt in canine pulmonary edema? J Appl Physiol Respir Environ Exerc Physiol 1984;57(4):1002–10.

40. Mansfield DR, Gollogly NC, Kaye DM, et al. Controlled trial of continuous positive airway pressure in obstructive sleep apnea and heart failure. Am J Respir Crit Care Med 2004;169(3):361–6.

41. Egea CJ, Aizpuru F, Pinto JA, et al. Cardiac function after CPAP therapy in patients with chronic heart failure and sleep apnea: a multicenter study. Sleep Med 2008;9(6):660–6.

42. Smith LA, Vennelle M, Gardner RS, et al. Auto-titrating continuous positive airway pressure therapy in patients with chronic heart failure and obstructive sleep apnoea: a randomized placebo-controlled trial. Eur Heart J 2007;28(10):1221–7.

43. Javaheri S, Caref EB, Chen E, et al. Sleep apnea testing and outcomes in a large cohort of Medicare beneficiaries with newly diagnosed heart failure. Am J Respir Crit Care Med 2011;183(4):539–46.

44. Kasai T, Narui K, Dohi T, et al. Prognosis of patients with heart failure and obstructive sleep apnea treated with continuous positive airway pressure. Chest 2008;133(3):690–6.

45. Wellman A, Malhotra A, Fogel RB, et al. Respiratory system loop gain in normal men and women measured with proportional-assist ventilation. J Appl Physiol 2003;94(1):205–12.

46. Randerath W. Sleep and heart. In: Chokroverty S, Ferini-Strambi L, editors. Sleep and its disorders. Oxford (United Kingdom): Oxford University Press; in press.

47. Randerath W, Khayat R, Arzt M, et al. Missing links. Sleep Med 2015;16(12):1495–6.

48. Solin P, Bergin P, Richardson M, et al. Influence of pulmonary capillary wedge pressure on central apnea in heart failure. Circulation 1999;99(12):1574–9.

49. Randerath W. Central and mixed sleep-related breathing disorders. In: Barkoukis T, Matheson J, Ferber R, et al, editors. Therapy in sleep medicine. Philadelphia: Elsevier; 2012. p. 243–53.

50. Wilcox I, McNamara SG, Dodd MJ, et al. Ventilatory control in patients with sleep apnoea and left ventricular dysfunction: comparison of obstructive and central sleep apnoea. Eur Respir J 1998;11(1):7–13.

51. Carmona-Bernal C, Quintana-Gallego E, Villa-Gil M, et al. Brain natriuretic peptide in patients with congestive heart failure and central sleep apnea. Chest 2005;127(5):1667–73.

52. Solin P, Kaye DM, Little PJ, et al. Impact of sleep apnea on sympathetic nervous system activity in heart failure. Chest 2003;123(4):1119–26.

53. Bitter T, Westerheide N, Prinz C, et al. Cheyne-Stokes respiration and obstructive sleep apnoea

are independent risk factors for malignant ventricular arrhythmias requiring appropriate cardioverter-defibrillator therapies in patients with congestive heart failure. Eur Heart J 2011;32(1):61–74.

54. Javaheri S, Shukla R, Wexler L. Association of smoking, sleep apnea, and plasma alkalosis with nocturnal ventricular arrhythmias in men with systolic heart failure. Chest 2012;141(6):1449–56.

55. Javaheri S, Shukla R, Zeigler H, et al. Central sleep apnea, right ventricular dysfunction, and low diastolic blood pressure are predictors of mortality in systolic heart failure. J Am Coll Cardiol 2007; 49(20):2028–34.

56. Javaheri S, Corbett WS. Association of low PaCO2 with central sleep apnea and ventricular arrhythmias in ambulatory patients with stable heart failure. Ann Intern Med 1998;128(3):204–7.

57. Randerath W, Verbraecken J, Andreas S, et al. Definition, discrimination, diagnosis and treatment of central breathing disturbances during sleep. Eur Respir J 2017;49(1).

58. Aurora RN, Chowdhuri S, Ramar K, et al. The treatment of central sleep apnea syndromes in adults: practice parameters with an evidence-based literature review and meta-analyses. Sleep 2012;35(1): 17–40.

59. Bradley TD, Logan AG, Kimoff RJ, et al. Continuous positive airway pressure for central sleep apnea and heart failure. N Engl J Med 2005;353(19): 2025–33.

60. Arzt M, Floras JS, Logan AG, et al. Suppression of central sleep apnea by continuous positive airway pressure and transplant-free survival in heart failure: a post hoc analysis of the Canadian Continuous Positive Airway Pressure for Patients with Central Sleep Apnea and Heart Failure Trial (CANPAP). Circulation 2007;115(25):3173–80.

61. Sands SA, Edwards BA, Kee K, et al. Loop gain as a means to predict a positive airway pressure suppression of Cheyne-Stokes respiration in patients with heart failure. Am J Respir Crit Care Med 2011; 184(9):1067–75.

62. Javaheri S, Brown LK, Randerath WJ. Positive airway pressure therapy with adaptive servoventilation: part 1: operational algorithms. Chest 2014; 146(2):514–23.

63. Javaheri S, Brown LK, Randerath WJ. Clinical applications of adaptive servoventilation devices: part 2. Chest 2014;146(3):858–68.

64. Javaheri S, Goetting MG, Khayat R, et al. The performance of two automatic servo-ventilation devices in the treatment of central sleep apnea. Sleep 2011; 34(12):1693–8.

65. Randerath WJ, Galetke W, Stieglitz S, et al. Adaptive servo-ventilation in patients with coexisting obstructive sleep apnoea/hypopnoea and Cheyne-Stokes respiration. Sleep Med 2008;9(8):823–30.

66. Randerath WJ, Galetke W, Kenter M, et al. Combined adaptive servo-ventilation and automatic positive airway pressure (anticyclic modulated ventilation) in co-existing obstructive and central sleep apnea syndrome and periodic breathing. Sleep Med 2009;10(8):898–903.

67. Randerath WJ, Nothofer G, Priegnitz C, et al. Long-term auto servo-ventilation or constant positive pressure in heart failure and co-existing central with obstructive sleep apnea. Chest 2012;142(2):440–7.

68. Dellweg D, Kerl J, Hoehn E, et al. Randomized controlled trial of noninvasive positive pressure ventilation (NPPV) versus servoventilation in patients with CPAP-induced central sleep apnea (complex sleep apnea). Sleep 2013;36(8):1163–71.

69. Javaheri S, Randerath W. Opioids-induced central sleep apnea: mechanisms and therapies. Sleep Med Clin 2014;9:49–56.

70. Javaheri S, Harris N, Howard J, et al. Adaptive servoventilation for treatment of opioid-associated central sleep apnea. J Clin Sleep Med 2014; 10(6):637–43.

71. Oldenburg O, Bitter T, Lehmann R, et al. Adaptive servoventilation improves cardiac function and respiratory stability. Clin Res Cardiol 2011;100(2): 107–15.

72. Kazimierczak A, Krzyzanowski K, Wierzbowski R, et al. Resolution of exercise oscillatory ventilation with adaptive servoventilation in patients with chronic heart failure and Cheyne-Stokes respiration: preliminary study. Kardiol Pol 2011;69(12): 1266–71.

73. Pepperell JC, Maskell NA, Jones DR, et al. A randomized controlled trial of adaptive ventilation for Cheyne-Stokes breathing in heart failure. Am J Respir Crit Care Med 2003;168(9):1109–14.

74. Sharma BK, Bakker JP, McSharry DG, et al. Adaptive servoventilation for treatment of sleep-disordered breathing in heart failure: a systematic review and meta-analysis. Chest 2012;142(5):1211–21.

75. Galetke W, Ghassemi BM, Priegnitz C, et al. Anticyclic modulated ventilation versus continuous positive airway pressure in patients with coexisting obstructive sleep apnea and Cheyne-Stokes respiration: a randomized crossover trial. Sleep Med 2014;15(8):874–9.

76. Momomura S, Seino Y, Kihara Y, et al. Adaptive servo-ventilation therapy for patients with chronic heart failure in a confirmatory, multicenter, randomized, controlled study. Circ J 2015;79(5):981–90.

77. Hetzenecker A, Escourrou P, Kuna ST, et al. Treatment of sleep apnea in chronic heart failure patients with auto-servo ventilation improves sleep fragmentation: a randomized controlled trial. Sleep Med 2016;17:25–31.

78. Hetzenecker A, Roth T, Birner C, et al. Adaptive servo-ventilation therapy of central sleep apnoea

and its effect on sleep quality. Clin Res Cardiol 2016; 105(3):189–95.

79. Toyama T, Hoshizaki H, Kasama S, et al. Adaptive servo-ventilation therapy improves cardiac sympathetic nerve activity, cardiac function, exercise capacity, and symptom in patients with chronic heart failure and Cheyne-Stokes respiration. J Nucl Cardiol 2016. [Epub ahead of print].

80. Takama N, Kurabayashi M. Effect of adaptive servo-ventilation on 1-year prognosis in heart failure patients. Circ J 2012;76(3):661–7.

81. Eulenburg C, Wegscheider K, Woehrle H, et al. Mechanisms underlying increased mortality risk in patients with heart failure and reduced ejection fraction randomly assigned to adaptive servoventilation in the SERVE-HF study: results of a secondary multistate modelling analysis. Lancet Respir Med 2016; 4(11):873–81.

82. Javaheri S, Brown L, Randerath W, et al. SERVE-HF: more questions than answers. Chest 2016; 149:900–4.

83. Lenique F, Habis M, Lofaso F, et al. Ventilatory and hemodynamic effects of continuous positive airway pressure in left heart failure. Am J Respir Crit Care Med 1997;155(2):500–5.

84. Tkacova R, Rankin F, Fitzgerald FS, et al. Effects of continuous positive airway pressure on obstructive sleep apnea and left ventricular afterload in patients with heart failure. Circulation 1998; 98(21):2269–75.

85. Spiesshofer J, Fox H, Lehmann R, et al. Heterogenous haemodynamic effects of adaptive servo-ventilation therapy in sleeping patients with heart failure and Cheyne-Stokes respiration compared to healthy volunteers. Heart Vessels 2015;31(7): 1117–30.

Non–Mask-based Therapies for Central Sleep Apnea in Patients with Heart Failure

Robin Germany, MD

KEYWORDS

- Central sleep apnea • Heart failure • Phrenic nerve stimulation • Theophylline • Acetazolamide
- Cardiac resynchronization thereapy

KEY POINTS

- Central sleep apnea (CSA) is highly prevalent in the heart failure (HF) population.
- Untreated CSA increases HF hospitalization and mortality.
- Treatments are limited currently to oxygen and positive airway pressure (PAP), which suffer from compliance issues and lack of randomized long-term data.
- Neurostimulation of the phrenic nerve offers a new therapeutic approach to treat CSA.

INTRODUCTION

CSA affects approximately one-third of patients with HF and is characterized by periods of shallow or absent breathing followed by periods of rapid, deep breathing (**Fig. 1**).[1,2] CSA results from a failure of the brain to appropriately recognize and respond to changes in carbon dioxide resulting in a cyclic breathing pattern.[3] CSA is uniquely tied to HF; HF can cause CSA and CSA can worsen HF resulting in increased mortality.[1] This inter-relationship requires that both parts of the cardio-sleep syndrome must be treated for either to improve. Identification of CSA is now simple and can often be done at home. A high index of suspicion is needed because patients present differently than the more common obstructive sleep apnea (OSA).

Although CSA has long-term detrimental effects, few treatment options are currently available. Oxygen, inhaled carbon dioxide, and medications have shown short-term benefit but lack any long-term randomized data.[4–6] PAP therapies have been the primary therapeutic option, but questions have been raised in light of data from recent trials.[7,8] A newer treatment based on neurostimulation of the phrenic nerve has recently published a large randomized trial and represents a new therapeutic option for patients with CSA.[9]

Because the cardio-sleep syndrome involves both the cardiologist and the sleep physician, it is of growing importance for the 2 specialties to work together to identify and treat patients with CSA. Continuing to develop an understanding regarding the inter-relationship of sleep and cardiovascular disease is important to identify the most appropriate therapeutic options for each patient.

PATHOPHYSIOLOGY

Each CSA cycle results in hypoxia and surges in sympathetic activity. Thus, each apnea-hyperpnea cycle contributes significant stress on the body, including disturbed sleep, sympathetic nervous system activation, acute pulmonary and

Disclosure: R. Germany is the Chief Medical Officer of Respicardia, Inc.
Cardiovascular Division, University of Oklahoma College of Medicine, 800 Stanton L. Young Boulevard, Oklahoma City, OK 73104, USA
E-mail address: Robin-germany@ouhsc.edu

Sleep Med Clin 12 (2017) 255–264
http://dx.doi.org/10.1016/j.jsmc.2017.02.001
1556-407X/17/© 2017 Elsevier Inc. All rights reserved.

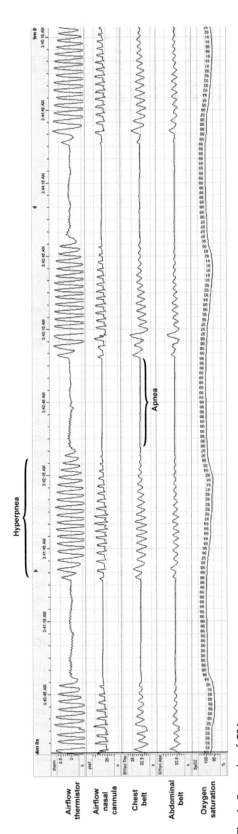

Fig. 1. Example of CSA.

systemic hypertension, plaque rupture, and arrhythmias.[3,10,11] As the cyclic breathing continues, these insults adversely affect the heart and contribute to the downward cycle of HF (**Fig. 2**).[3] In return, worsening HF increases sympathetic activation and fluid retention, contributing to the cyclic breathing pattern.[12] The result of this cardio-sleep syndrome is an increased risk for recurrent HF hospitalizations, ventricular arrhythmias, and death.[11,13–15]

CSA results in recurrent arousals associated with discrete increases in sympathetic drive.[16] These surges result in increased blood pressure, fluid retention, myocardial fibrosis, and peripheral vasoconstriction.[3] The consequences further lead to tachycardia and both ventricular and atrial arrhythmias.[11,17] In addition, this constant nightly elevation in sympathetic drive leads to progressive cardiac dysfunction and cardiovascular death.

Hypoxia also plays an important role in the pathophysiology of CSA and ties closely with long-term outcomes.[3] Hypoxia leads to myocardial ischemia and poor cerebral perfusion. Hypoxia also results in inflammation and endothelial dysfunction. In injured myocardium, elevations in inflammatory factors have an adverse impact on left ventricular function, contribute to pulmonary edema as well as to cachexia, and predict increased mortality in HF patients. There is a growing interest in hypoxia as the primary driver of the adverse effects of CSA, with 1 study showing hypoxia more predictive of mortality than AHI alone.[3]

There is an increasing appreciation for the affect CSA has on sleep quality. The recent American Heart Association/American College of Cardiology guidance document notes that poor outcomes are associated with less than 7 hours or more than 9 hours of sleep.[18] Poor sleep quality is associated with poor work performance, poor cognitive function, increased blood pressure, and increased cardiovascular events.[3,15,19] HF patients with CSA demonstrate a significant reduction in sleep time with an average of 4 hours to 5 hours.[20] The quality of sleep is also reduced with significant reductions in REM sleep and in restful sleep.[20]

The results of the long-term effect of CSA are evident when examining the outcomes of HF patients with CSA. Mortality remains at 50% at 5 years in the untreated CSA HF population compared with approximately 25% in HF patients without CSA.[13,14,21] CSA patients hospitalized with HF have a 50% readmission rate at 6 months and 25% have more than 1 hospitalization.[15] There is an increased rate of ventricular arrhythmias and appropriate implantable cardioverter defibrillator shocks in similar patients with CSA compared with those without.[11] CSA is clearly detrimental to patients and based on physiology, and reducing the amount of CSA experienced should lead to significant beneficial effects.

IDENTIFICATION OF CENTRAL SLEEP APNEA HEART FAILURE PATIENTS

CSA has traditionally been thought to occur primarily in the HF with reduced ejection fraction (HFrEF) population; however, it seems the prevalence is only slightly lower in the HF with preserved ejection fraction (HFpEF) population.[22] Although there was a range of prevalence in the HFrEF population in early studies, prevalence studies conducted following guideline-directed medical therapy for HF have been more consistent.[14,23,24] The largest prospective study in the HFrEF

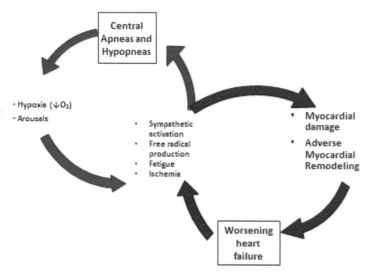

Fig. 2. The cardio-sleep syndrome. (*Adapted from* Bekfani T, Abraham WT. Current and future developments in the field of central sleep apnoea. Europace 2016;18(8):1127; with permission.)

population demonstrated that 40% of the 700 HFrEF patients had CSA.[23] Similarly, a less symptomatic patient population had a similar prevalence of CSA at 37%.[13] Although slightly lower, the prevalence in the HFpEF population remains at 31%.[22] There seems to be a slightly higher prevalence by lower ejection fraction or higher symptoms (increased New York Heart Association classification).[3] Therefore, a high index of suspicion is needed when evaluating an HF patient.

Although patients with HF and CSA have a significant reduction in sleep, they rarely complain about sleepiness.[25] It has been proposed that this is due to the increase in sympathetic drive already associated with HF, which may make patients feel fatigued rather than sleepy.[3] Many of the symptoms of CSA are similar to those experienced with HF, such as fatigue, poor mental focus, or gasping at night (**Box 1**). Patients with CSA may present with periodic breathing during the daytime or their partners may notice either disrupted or pauses in breathing at night.[3] Regardless, it is clear that traditional questionnaires to identify healthy patients with OSA do not work in HF patients for either CSA or OSA.[25]

Box 1
Signs and symptoms of central sleep apnea

Patients at high risk for CSA

- Recent HF hospitalization or symptomatic HF
- Atrial or ventricular arrhythmias
- Witnessed apneas
- Male
- Elderly
- Lean (nonobese)
- Decreased exercise tolerance
- Low ejection fraction
- Paroxysmal nocturnal dyspnea
- Stroke
- Carotid stenosis
- Diabetes mellitus
- Chronic fatigue
- Nocturia (>2 per night)

Data from Costanzo MR, Khayat R, Ponikowski P, et al. Mechanisms and clinical consequences of untreated central sleep apnea in heart failure. J Am Coll Cardiol 2015;65:72–84; and Khayat RN, Jarjoura D, Patt B, et al. In-hospital testing for sleep-disordered breathing in hospitalized patients with decompensated heart failure: report of prevalence and patient characteristics. J Card Fail 2009;15:739–46.

CSA traditionally has been diagnosed through polysomnography (PSG) performed in a sleep laboratory with a sleep technician in attendance. Based on current guidelines, the PSG is diagnostic for CSA if respiratory monitoring demonstrates at least 3 consecutive cycles of crescendo-decrescendo change in breathing amplitude and 1 or both of the following: (1) 5 or more CSA or hypopneas per sleep hour and/or (2) cyclic crescendo-decrescendo breathing for greater than or equal to 10 consecutive minutes. CSA severity commonly is described by the apnea-hypopnea index (AHI), defined as the number of apnea and hypopnea events per hour.[26] Although patients may have both CSA and OSA, the predominant form typically classifies the disorder.

Although many patients go to a sleep laboratory for diagnosis, portable sleep monitors are designed to be used in the home environment. Several different types of portable monitors are commercially available, with each device differing in the number and type of sleep-related variables they monitor. Level 3 portable monitors, which record at least 3 channels of data (eg, oximetry, airflow, and respiratory effort) demonstrate accurate diagnostic performance in patients and can distinguish obstructive from central events based on belt movement.[27] It is important to remember that these devices have a higher false-negative rate and can underestimate the severity of the disease due to the inability to identify sleep but allow testing of patients in their own home.

TREATMENT OPTIONS FOR CENTRAL SLEEP APNEA

Optimum treatment of CSA in HF patients is limited. Treatment typically begins with optimizing HF therapies, which may reduce the burden of CSA. After HF optimization, PAP therapies have traditionally been the mainstay of therapy; however, concerns have been raised recently due to the adverse outcomes in the recently published Treatment of Sleep-Disordered Breathing with Predominant Central Sleep Apnea by Adaptive Servo Ventilation in Patients with Heart Failure (SERVE-HF) study, as discussed in another article in this edition.[8] Phrenic nerve stimulation has now published its randomized clinical trial showing excellent compliance and strong clinical outcomes.[9] Oxygen has been used and improves symptoms in some studies, but no long-term randomized trials have been completed.[4] Other therapeutic options that have been considered either failed or have limited randomized or long-term data.[3] These therapeutic options include several medications, carbon dioxide, and atrial pacing.

Therefore, it is important to understand the data available on these therapeutic options.

Heart Failure Therapy Optimization

The treatment of CSA in HF patients begins with the optimization of HF therapies. Although early studies anticipated that CSA would resolve if the ejection fraction improved, it is now recognized that the development of CSA occurs via multiple mechanisms, which include, but are not limited to, increased sympathetic activation and ejection fraction. Thus, resolution or improvement of HF may not have a significant impact on the severity of CSA in all patients. Studies have demonstrated, however, a reduction in the number of events per hour with diuretics, angiotensin-converting enzyme inhibition, β-blockers, and cardiac resynchronization therapy. CRT therapy held the most promise to improve CSA with initial studies demonstrating significant resolution of CSA in symptomatic HF patients with a widen QRS on ECG (>120 ms) and an ejection fraction less than 35%.[28,29] CRT is now standard of care in appropriate patients, but prevalence studies continue to demonstrate approximately 35% of patients have CSA.[14] Studies prospectively following patients long term who initially improve after CRT implant would add to the literature and increase understanding of the appropriate time to screen patients after CRT. Although optimizing HF therapy is important, treating CSA as soon as possible is important to mitigate the continued insult from unabated hypoxia and sympathetic surges.

Few data exist on the treatment of patients awaiting left ventricular assist device and cardiac transplant. These patients have the most ominous cases of CSA but may achieve resolution after the procedure.[30,31] In addition, these are patient, who may be at higher risk from PAP therapies, especially if they have a low wedge pressure, because PAP therapies can decrease cardiac output in these severe cases.[32] Thus, research is clearly needed in this area.

Positive Airway Pressure Therapies

Positive airway therapies are a group of devices that blow air into the lungs to increase airflow similar to a ventilator. These therapies were initially designed to open closed airways in the treatment of OSA but were then used in CSA. Dr Randerath describes these therapies in detail (see Winfried Randerath and Simon Herkenrath's article, "Device Therapy for Sleep-Disordered Breathing in Patients with Cardiovascular Diseases and Heart Failure," in this issue). Briefly, CSA is currently treated primarily with PAP therapies.[33] Patients with CSA receiving PAP therapies have experienced improvement in AHI and cardiovascular variables but suffer from poor patient acceptance and compliance.[7] In a recent prospective study, 52% of patients either refused PAP therapy or were not compliant with the therapy.[34] The largest study to date in CSA patients demonstrated that at 1 year, 28% had stopped therapy and only 45% of the remaining patients (32% overall) used the therapy at least 3 hours per night, suggesting PAP therapy may not be a good long-term solution.[7]

There have been few randomized, multicenter trials using PAP therapies in the treatment of CSA and these have focused on HF patients with reduced ejection fraction. The largest randomized study using CPAP demonstrated an average reduction in AHI of 21 events per hour while the patient was using the therapy (on average 3.6 hours/night at 1 year). This trial, however, failed to meet its primary endpoint and raised concerns about the therapy due to an increased early mortality signal.[7]

A newer form of PAP therapy, adaptive servo-ventilation (ASV), was designed specifically for HF patients. ASV was designed to change pressures based on a patient's individual needs with the expectation that lower airway pressure would be delivered. The SERVE-HF, a multicenter, randomized controlled trial, was designed to assess whether the treatment of moderate to severe CSA with ASV therapy could reduce mortality and morbidity in patients with symptomatic chronic HF (left ventricular ejection fraction [LVEF] ≤45%) in addition to optimized medical care.[8] The study failed to meet its primary endpoint of a reduction in cardiovascular morbidity and mortality. Furthermore, cardiovascular mortality was increased in patients in the ASV treatment arm compared with those in the control arm, with an absolute annual mortality rate of 10% vs 7.5%. This increase in mortality seems to be driven by an increase in cardiovascular deaths without a preceding HF hospitalization. The investigators proposed 2 reasons: (1) CSA may be a compensatory mechanism in patients with HF and (2) application of positive pressure may impair cardiac function in some patients. Although it has been hypothesized that CSA could be another compensatory mechanism in systolic HF, any benefits from CSA would be temporary and occur only in hyperventilatory phase of the cyclic breathing pattern. In addition, hyperventilatory effects would be augmented by ASV and should have resulted in a strongly positive ASV trial. The possible detrimental cardiac effects of PAP therapy in HFrEF patients with CSA also has been discussed in the literature. Even mildly elevated PAPs have been shown to result in acute negative hemodynamic effects, such as decreased cardiac output and hypotension in some HFrEF patients.[32] PAP could also lead to elevated right heart pressure contributing to progressive right ventricular dysfunction and sudden cardiac death, especially in patients with weakened right heart function due to underlying cardiac conditions. Regardless of the reason for the failed trial, ASV is now a class III contraindication in the HF guidelines for patients with an ejection fraction less than 45%.[35]

Oxygen

Supplemental nocturnal oxygen therapy at 2 L/min to 4 L/min by nasal cannula has been used to treat CSA in patients with HF. Data from several small, short-term studies have shown that oxygen improves the AHI and exercise capacity and reduces serum B-type natriuretic peptide levels and sympathetic nervous system activity.[4,36,37] It does not seem, however, to improve daytime sleepiness or cognitive function or to have any consistent effect on quality of life, LVEF, or sleep quality. The longest studies using oxygen for CSA have been approximately 3 months long and continued to lack any benefit in quality of life.[38,39] No long-term or large-scale randomized trials have been completed and questions have been raised about the possibility of harmful effects of oxygen therapy in HF due to the detrimental effects of hyperoxia, including vasoconstriction in both the coronary and cerebral vascular beds.[40]

Oxygen is not recommended routinely in HF patients without CSA because it has been shown to decrease cardiac index and increase infarct size post–myocardial infarction.[40] Currently, HF guidelines only recommend oxygen for patients hypoxemic at rest (1C recommendation, Heart Failure Society of America) and against oxygen for patient with normal baseline oxygen levels (class III recommendation).[41] The recently published European Society of Cardiology HF guidelines (2016) remain silent on oxygen at night for the treatment of CSA.[42] In the 2012 American Academy of Sleep Medicine recommendations, oxygen was considered an appropriate therapy based on several small studies showing possible benefit and lack of harm.[33] Thus, there is no consistent recommendation on the use of oxygen for the treatment of CSA.

Phrenic Nerve Stimulation

A new device that delivers neurostimulation to the phrenic nerve (remedē System, Respicardia, Minnetonka, Minnesota) (**Fig. 3**) was developed to restore and stabilize the breathing pattern of patients with CSA by contraction of the diaphragm similar to normal breathing. Neurostimulation of the phrenic nerve was designed to eliminate patient compliance/adherence issues by activating automatically and removing the need for patient interaction or adherence. The neurostimulation system stimulates a single phrenic nerve, producing changes in carbon dioxide levels and tidal volumes similar to normal breathing.[43] It is implanted in the cardiac suite with a transvenous stimulation lead implanted either into the left pericardiophrenic or the right brachiocephalic vein. A sensing lead is implanted into a branch of the azygous vein and the device is placed into either the right or left pectoral area. The device provides neurostimulation pulses configured to smoothly engage the diaphragm similar to normal breathing (**Fig. 4**).[44]

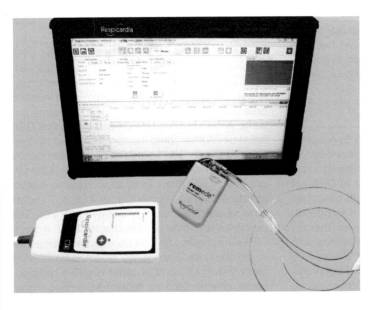

Fig. 3. The remedē System: neurostimulation of the phrenic nerve. CAUTION Investigational device. Limited by federal (or United States) law to investigational use. (*Courtesy of* Respicardia, Minnetonka, MN; with permission.)

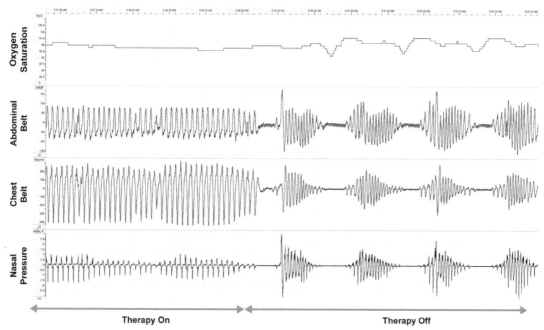

Fig. 4. Effects of neurostimulation of the phrenic nerve on the breathing pattern.

A prospective, multicenter, nonrandomized pilot study was completed in patients with moderate to severe CSA; 57 patients were enrolled and followed for 3 months. Neurostimulation of the phrenic nerve improved AHI, central apnea index, oxygen desaturation index, arousals, and rapid eye movement sleep; 45% of patients reported moderate to marked improvement in quality of life by patient global assessment and Minnesota Living with Heart Failure score by an average of 10 points in patients with HF (P<.001).[45]

After the pilot study, neurostimulation of the phrenic nerve was studied in a large randomized, multicenter study with blinded endpoint assessment.[44] The study was not restricted to HF patients, but 66% of subjects did have HF. A full-night PSG was completed to assess primary effectiveness: comparison of the proportions of treatment versus control patients achieving a greater than or equal to 50% AHI reduction, determined by a blinded PSG core laboratory. The primary safety endpoint of 12-month freedom from procedural-related, system-related, or therapy-related serious adverse events was evaluated in all patients; 151 patients with moderate to severe CSA were randomized. A higher proportion of patients in the treatment group had an AHI reduction greater than or equal to 50% at 6 months compared with controls (51% vs 11%, P<.0001), in the intention-to-treat analysis population; 12-month freedom from procedure-related, device-related, or therapy-related serious adverse

events was 91%. Significant improvements were noted in oxygen desaturation index, arousals, and rapid eye movement sleep; 60% of subjects reported moderate or marked improvement in patient global assessment, and the Epworth Sleepiness Scale improved by 3.7 points (P<.001 between groups).[45] Neurostimulation of the phrenic nerve offers an exciting new therapeutic option for patients with CSA.

Additional Therapeutic Concepts

Several other therapeutic ideas have been studied for the treatment of CSA. There is a lack of data or documented beneficial effect, however, to many of them. Reviewing the data does allow insight into the mechanisms involved in the disease process and may lead to the development of other therapeutic options.

Medications

Although several medications have been tested for CSA, none has been tested in large randomized studies and none is currently approved for the treatment of CSA. These medical trials have helped confirm, however, the role of carbon dioxide metabolism in cyclic breathing and are included in this review for completeness. Acetazolamide is a mild diuretic agent causing metabolic acidosis resulting in a decreased $Paco_2$, which increases the level of $Paco_2$ needed to cause an apnea. In a single, double-blind study, acetazolamide showed improvement in subjective sleep quality and decreased both the respiratory events and nocturnal oxygen desaturation.[46] It did not show any improvement, however, in LVEF or in the objective measurement of sleep quality. In addition, the use of acetazolamide causes urinary potassium wasting, which could lead to arrhythmias. Therefore, the use of acetazolamide in treating patients with HF and CSA is not recommended currently. Benzodiazepines can reduce arousability and 1 small study examined whether CSA could be decreased by decreasing arousals and thus the ventilator overshoot leading to CSR. The study did show a decrease in microarousals but failed to show an improvement in time in CSR or time below 90%.[47] Theophylline, as a respiratory stimulant, has been proposed for the treatment of CSA in HF. Therapeutic effect may involve increased ventilatory responsiveness below eupnea, resulting in increased proximity between eupneic $Paco_2$ and the apnea threshold. In 1 small, short-term study of patients with CSA and stable HF, compared with placebo, theophylline decreased central apnea and oxyhemoglobin desaturation.[48] Theophylline is associated with ventricular arrhythmias, thus limiting the use of this medication in the HF population.[49] Thus, currently there is no medication demonstrated to have an impact on CSA long term.

Supplemental carbon dioxide

Changes in carbon dioxide above and below the apneic threshold drive CSA. Due to the delay in recognizing these changes, hyperventilation results in driving the CO_2 level well below the apneic threshold. Thus, supplemental CO_2 could theoretically stabilize the breathing pattern by increasing baseline ventilation and increasing the difference between the baseline $Paco_2$ and the apnea threshold. Increasing baseline CO_2 has been studied using 2 different methodologies: dead-space breathing and inhaled CO_2.[5,50] An increase in dead space using a cylinder of air in 8 patients with CSA demonstrated improvements in apneas and arousals.[50] No further work has been done, however, in this area.

Inhaled carbon dioxide has been studied with 2 different methodologies. Initial work with inhaled carbon dioxide demonstrated a reduction in apneas and hypopneas but resulted in increased respiratory rate and increases the work of breathing thought to be detrimental in HF.[5] After this, dynamic carbon dioxide (given at the peak of hyperventilation) was given to 7 healthy individuals during voluntary hyperventilation and was found to inhibit the oscillatory breathing response.[51] To date, however, neither methodology has been

studied on a large scale. There are no trials to support use in HF patients to date. In addition, patient safety and therapeutic delivery remain a significant challenge. Thus, supplemental carbon dioxide is not currently recommended to treat CSA in HF.

Atrial pacing

Although CRT is part of the normal treatment of patients with HF and reduced ejection fraction, a group of investigators found that pacing patients with CSA in the atrium at a rate 10 beats higher per minute than baseline improved apnea and hypopneic events.[52] This could be due to the temporary improvement in cardiac output with increase heart rate. It was unclear, however, if this was an acute reaction only and no long-term study has been published to date. In addition, it is now recognized that a lower heart rate is beneficial in HFrEF patients and thus it is unexpected that this therapy will be developed further.[53]

SUMMARY

CSA affects approximately 1 in 3 HF patients, increasing the risk for hospitalization and death. Although CSA has important detrimental effects on the cardiovascular system, HF in turn can trigger or worsen CSA making it important to treat both parts of the cardio-sleep syndrome. With the high prevalence, patients are easy to identify either in a sleep laboratory or with home testing. The difficulty to date has been the few therapeutic options available to treat CSA. Currently, continuous PAP is the most common option but is limited by patient acceptance and concern about PAP in some patients with reduced ejection fraction. Oxygen has also been recommended but needs additional research due to the lack of long-term data and in light of the detrimental effects of hyperoxia. Neurostimulation of the phrenic nerve is an exciting new therapeutic approach that will add significantly to the therapeutic options for CSA. The field of CSA continues to grow in importance as new therapeutic options arise and treat this devastating disease.

REFERENCES

1. Brenner S, Angermann C, Berthold J, et al. Sleep-disordered breathing and heart failure: a dangerous liaison. Trends Cardiovasc Med 2008;18:240–7.
2. Javaheri S, Dempsey JA. Central sleep apnea. Compr Physiol 2013;3:141–63.
3. Costanzo MR, Khayat R, Ponikowski P, et al. State-of-the-art review: mechanisms and clinical consequences of untreated central sleep apnea in heart failure. J Am Coll Cardiol 2015;65:72–84.

4. Franklin K, Eriksson P, Sahlin C, et al. Reversal of central sleep apnea with oxygen. Chest 1997;111: 163–9.

5. Lorenzi-Filho G, Rankin F, Bies I, et al. Effects of inhaled carbon dioxide and oxygen on Cheyne-Stokes Respiration in patients with heart failure. Am J Respir Crit Care Med 1999;159:1490–9.

6. Khayat R, Abraham WT. Current treatment approaches and trials in central sleep apnea. Int J Cardiol 2016;206:S22–7.

7. Bradley TD, Logan AG, Kimoff RJ, et al. Continuous positive airway pressure for central sleep apnea and heart failure. N Engl J Med 2005;353(19):2025–33.

8. Cowie MR, Hoehrle H, Wegscheider K, et al. Adaptive servo-ventilation for central sleep apnea in systolic heart failure. N Engl J Med 2015;373:1095–105.

9. Costanzo MR, Ponikowski P, Javaheri S, et al. Randomised controlled trial of transvenous neurostimulation for central sleep apnoea. Lancet 2016;388:974–82.

10. Dempsey JA, Veasey SC, Morgan BJ, et al. Pathophysiology of sleep apnea. Physiol Rev 2010;90: 47–112.

11. Bitter T, Westerheide N, Prinz C, et al. Cheyne-Stokes respiration and obstructive sleep apnoea are independent risk factors for malignant ventricular arrhythmias requiring appropriate cardioverter-defibrillator therapies in patients with congestive heart failure. Eur Heart J 2011;32:61–74.

12. Floras JS. Sympathetic nervous system activation in human heart failure. J Am Coll Cardiol 2009;54:375–85.

13. Javaheri S. Sleep disorders in systolic heart failure: a prospective study of 100 male patients. The final report. Int J Cardiol 2006;106:21–8.

14. Jilek C, Krenn M, Sebah, et al. Prognostic impact of sleep disordered breathing and its treatment in heart failure: an observational study. Eur J Heart Fail 2011; 13:68–75.

15. Khayat R, Abraham W, Patt B, et al. Central sleep apnea is a predictor of cardiac readmission in hospitalized patients with systolic heart failure. J Card Fail 2012;18:534–40.

16. Somers VK, Dyken ME, Mark AL, et al. Sympathetic-nerve activity during sleep in normal subjects. N Engl J Med 1993;328:303–7.

17. Leung RST, Huber MA, Rogge T, et al. Association between atrial fibrillation and central sleep apnea. Sleep 2005;28(12):1543–6.

18. St-Onge MP, Grandner MA, Brown D, et al. Sleep duration and quality: impact on lifestyle behavior and cardiometabolic health. Circulation 2016; 134(18):e367–86.

19. Yaffe K, Laffan AM, Harrison SL, et al. Sleep-disordered breathing, hypoxia, and risk of mild cognitive impairment and dementia in older women. JAMA 2011;306:613–9.

20. Javaheri S, Parker TJ, Liming JD, et al. Sleep apnea in 81 ambulatory male patients with stable heart failure: types and their prevalences, consequences, and presentations. Circulation 1998;97:2154–9.

21. Khayat R, Jarjoura D, Porter K, et al. Sleep disordered breathing and post-discharge mortality in patients with acute heart failure. Eur Heart J 2015; 36(23):1463–9.

22. Bitter T, Faber L, Hering D, et al. Sleep-disordered breathing in heart failure with normal left ventricular ejection fraction. Eur J Heart Fail 2009;11:602–8.

23. Oldenburg O, Lamp B, Faber L, et al. Sleep-disordered breathing in patients with symptomatic heart failure. A contemporary study of prevalence in and characteristics of 700 patients. Eur J Heart Fail 2007;9:251–7.

24. Arzt M, Woehrle H, Oldenburg O, et al. Prevalence and predictors of sleep-disordered breathing in patients with stable chronic heart failure: the SchlaHF registry. JACC Heart Fail 2016;4:116–25.

25. Hastings PC, Vazir A, O'Driscoll DM, et al. Symptom burden of sleep-disordered breathing in mild-to-moderate congestive heart failure patients. Eur Respir J 2006;27:748–55.

26. Iber C, Ancoli-Israel S, Chesson AL Jr, et al, for the American Academy of Sleep Medicine. The AASM manual for the scoring of sleep and associated events: rules, terminology and technical specifications. Westchester (IL): American Academy of Sleep Medicine; 2007.

27. Cairns A, Wickwire E, Schaefer E, et al. A pilot validation study for the NOX T3 portable monitor for the detection for OSA. Sleep Breath 2014;18:609–14.

28. Skobel EC, Sinha AM, Norra C, et al. Effect of cardiac resynchronization therapy on sleep quality, quality of life and symptomatic depression in patients with chronic heart failure and Cheyne-Stokes respiration. Sleep Breath 2005;9:159–66.

29. Sinha AM, Skobel EC, Breithardt OA, et al. Cardiac resynchronization therapy improves central sleep apnea and Cheyne-Stokes respiration in patients with chronic heart failure. J Am Coll Cardiol 2004;44:68–71.

30. Braver HM, Brandes WC, Kubiet MA, et al. Effect of cardiac transplant on Cheyne-Stokes respiration occurring during sleep. Am J Cardiol 1995;76:632–3.

31. Mansfield DR, Solin P, Roebuck T, et al. The effect of successful heart transplant treatment of heart failure on central sleep apnea. Chest 2003;124:1675–81.

32. Bradley TD, Holloway RM, McLaughlin PR, et al. Cardiac output response to continuous positive airway pressure in congestive heart failure. Am Rev Respir Dis 1992;145:377–82.

33. Aurora RN, Chowdhuri S, Ramar K, et al. The treatment of central sleep apnea syndromes in adults: practice parameters with and evidence based literature review and meta-analyses. Sleep 2012; 35:17–40.

34. Oldenburg O, Schmidt A, Lamp B, et al. Adaptive servoventilation improves cardiac function in

patients with chronic heart failure and Cheyne-Stokes respiration. Eur J Heart Fail 2008;10:581–6.

35. Aurora RN, Bist SR, Casey KR, et al. Updated adaptive servo-ventilation recommendation for the 2012 AASM Guidelines: "The treatment of central sleep apnea syndromes in adults: practice parameters with and evidence-based literature review and meta-analysis. J Clin Sleep Med 2016;12:757–61.

36. Javaheri S, Ahmed M, Parker T, et al. Effects of nasal O2 on sleep-related disordered breathing in ambulatory patients with stable heart failure. Sleep 1999; 22:1101–6.

37. Toyama T, Seki R, Kasama S, et al. Effectiveness of nocturnal home oxygen therapy to improve exercise capacity, cardiac function and cardiac sympathetic nerve activity in patients with chronic heart failure and central sleep apnea. Circ J 2009;73:299–304.

38. Krachman S, Nugent T, Crocetti J, et al. Effects of oxygen therapy on left ventricular function in patients with Cheyne-Stokes respiration and congestive heart failure. J Clin Sleep Med 2005;1:271–6.

39. Staniforth A, Kinnear W, Starling R, et al. Effect of oxygen on sleep quality, cognitive function, and sympathetic activity in patients with chronic heart failure and Cheyne-Stokes respiration. Eur Heart J 1998;19:922–8.

40. Sephrvand N, Ezekowitz JA. Oxygen therapy in patients with acute heart failure. JACC Heart Fail 2016; 4:783–90.

41. Albert NM, Boehmer JP, Collins SP, et al. HFSA 2010 Comprehensive heart failure practice guidelines. J Card Fail 2010;16:e1–94.

42. Ponikowski P, Voors AA, Anker SD, et al. 2016 ESC Guidelines for the diagnosis and treatment of acute and chronic heart failure. Rev Esp Cardiol (Engl Ed) 2016;69(12):1167.

43. Zhang X, Ding N, Ni B, et al. Safety and feasibility of chronic transvenous phrenic nerve stimulation for treatment of central sleep apnea in heart failure patients. Clin Respir J 2017;11(2):176–84.

44. Costanzo MR, Augostini R, Goldberg LR, et al. Design of the remedē® system pivotal trial: a prospective, randomized study in the use of respiratory rhythm management to treat central sleep apnea. J Card Fail 2015;21:892–902.

45. Abraham WT, Jagielski D, Oldenburg O, et al. Phrenic nerve stimulation for the treatment of central sleep apnea. JACC Heart Fail 2015;5:360–9.

46. Javaheri S. Acetazolamide improves central sleep apnea in heart failure. A double-blind, prospective study. Am J Respir Crit Care Med 2006;173: 234–7.

47. Biberdorf DJ, Steens R, Millar TW, et al. Benzodiazepines in congestive heart failure: effects of temazepam on arousability and Cheyne-Stokes Respiration. Sleep 1993;16:529–38.

48. Javaheri S, Parker TJ, Wexler L, et al. Effect of theophylline on sleep-disordered breathing in heart failure. N Engl J Med 1996;335:562–7.

49. Bittar G, Friedman HS. The arrhythmogenicity of theophylline. A multivariate analysis of clinical determinants. Chest 1991;99:1415–20.

50. Khayat RN, Xie A, Patel AK, et al. Cardiorespiratory effects of added dead space in patients with heart failure and central sleep apnea. Chest 2003;123: 1551–60.

51. Giannoni A, Baruah R, Wilson K, et al. Real-time dynamic carbon dioxide administration. J Am Coll Cardiol 2010;56:1832–7.

52. Garrigue S, Bordier P, Jais P, et al. Benefit of atrial pacing in sleep apnea syndrome. N Engl J Med 2002;346:404–12.

53. Dobre D, Borer JS, Fox K, et al. Heart rate: a prognostic factor and therapeutic target in chronic heart failure. The distinct roles of drugs with heart rate-lowering properties. Eur J Heart Fail 2014;16:76–85.

Moving?

Make sure your subscription moves with you!

To notify us of your new address, find your **Clinics Account Number** (located on your mailing label above your name), and contact customer service at:

Email: journalscustomerservice-usa@elsevier.com

800-654-2452 (subscribers in the U.S. & Canada)
314-447-8871 (subscribers outside of the U.S. & Canada)

Fax number: 314-447-8029

Elsevier Health Sciences Division
Subscription Customer Service
3251 Riverport Lane
Maryland Heights, MO 63043

*To ensure uninterrupted delivery of your subscription, please notify us at least 4 weeks in advance of move.

Printed and bound by CPI Group (UK) Ltd, Croydon, CR0 4YY

03/10/2024

01040304-0003